Prepared Childbirth
The Family Way

Throughout life we prepare for the things that really matter – school, career, marriage. Giving birth should be no exception. Because the birth event profoundly affects everyone involved, it deserves careful and thoughtful preparation. This manual was written to assist you in preparing for the birth of your child by reviewing material presented by your childbirth educator and offering guidelines for planning your birth. It reflects our philosophy that:

- childbirth is a joyful experience for which parents should prepare, and

- preparation should give a woman confidence in her body's ability to give birth, to nourish and nurture her children.

As your knowledge increases, discussions about alternatives regarding labor and birth become more meaningful. Soon you will be able to make informed decisions as you plan your approach to childbirth.

This is *Prepared Childbirth – The Family Way*

by

Debby Amis and Jeanne Green

For additional copies of this handbook, contact:

The Family Way Publications, Inc.

Phone: (713) 528-0277
Fax: (713) 583-6187
Website: www.thefamilyway.com
E-mail: info@thefamilyway.com

ISBN 0-9769758-9-0

Prepared Childbirth - The Family Way provides information of a general nature to accompany childbirth preparation classes. As medical circumstances can vary widely from woman to woman and time to time, each mother, father, baby, and setting presents a unique situation. This handbook is not designed to provide specific medical advice for any individual pregnancy or problem. Such individual advice is best obtained from the healthcare provider.

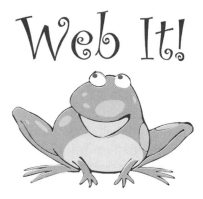

When you see this icon on a page, go to our website at **www.thefamilyway.com.** Click on the **Web It!** tab. Here you will find links to websites with reliable information on the topics indicated.

Preface

Prepared Childbirth - The Family Way was originally written to provide a state-of-the-art handbook for the classes taught by The Family Way, Inc. Since our first edition we have continued to keep up with current childbirth research and evidence-based practices, so that educators and parents-to-be can always depend upon this manual to be current, concise, and complete. While this handbook is not designed to substitute for trained medical advice and professional care, regular updates show our dedication to providing the best resource possible for educators and new parents. We welcome your comments and suggestions for this manual.

In this eighth edition we introduced the Web It! feature to expand your learning opportunities beyond the pages of this book and direct you to reliable sites on the Web.

In Appreciation

If it were not for the volunteer efforts of Linda and Tom Arnold, who were attending our classes when this book was just our dream, *Prepared Childbirth - The Family Way* might never have been published. Their patience and untiring efforts in the many revisions made the publication of our first edition possible. Two other very special people, Jo Ann Moffitt, RN, and Vicki Mullen, PT, coauthors in our original publication, have our deepest thanks. Both of them have moved on to other endeavors in their respective fields, but we will always be appreciative of the energy and knowledge they shared with us.

For hours of consultation and review of the breastfeeding section, we thank Jeannette Crenshaw, MSN, IBCLC. We also appreciate the review of Emergency Birth by Debbie Young, CD(DONA), EMT. We would like to acknowledge the contributions of our talented artists: Vicki Wright and Vonette Thorner drew the illustrations for the exercise and second-stage positions, and Stephen Brown prepared the outstanding anatomical illustrations. Bob Mader provided the beautiful photographic images of models Tina and Tomas Molander, Mackenzie Wheatly photographed Jordan and Brian Amis, and Joe Farrier contributed the photographs of Elaine and Gerard Boehme and Ashley Burgos-Cruz. We also thank Margie Wallis, Nicole Allman, Tommie Black, Christy and Andrew McWhorter, and Sheetal and Milind Joshi for appearing as models in our book.

We are grateful to our husbands, who have truly made this a family-centered business. Steve Amis has been invaluable in designing the layout of our book so that revisions and updates can be easily accomplished. Gordon Green has shared his proofreading and editing skills as well as his medical expertise on care of the newborn.

The parents whose birth reports we feature contributed much to the spirit of this book. A special thank-you to all the wonderful childbirth educators we have worked with and learned from over the years - locally through The Family Way, and internationally through Lamaze International, the International Childbirth Education Association, and DONA International. Lastly, we would like to thank the families in our childbirth classes who have shared their concerns, questions, tears, and joys of pregnancy and birth with us in The Family Way.

Who Are We?

Debby Amis: When I went off to college in Colorado, I wanted to be an international diplomat and solve the problems of the world. I took Russian, geography, and political science. Then Steve proposed and I realized that nursing or teaching would be more practical for putting him through law school. We both transferred from the University of Colorado to the University of Texas to complete our educations. During nursing school, I worked part-time in Labor and Delivery at Brackenridge Hospital in Austin. I was both fascinated with birth and horrified at having to strap down the women who chose Twilight Sleep. When I went home for the holidays, my OB dad would wake me so that I could accompany him to the births of the women who planned natural births. In the early 70s, Dad was featured in a TV news story as one of the few OBs in the Dallas area who would allow fathers into the delivery room.

After I spent several years nursing, both in the hospital and in public health, Steve graduated from law school. Six months later our first son, Brian, was born. Teaching childbirth classes seemed like the natural next step. I became certified by Lamaze International and active with a local community-based childbirth group. I had a second son, Ben. The rest, as they say, is history. I volunteered with Lamaze International and have continued to be an active member for many years. I have served as president and as Education Council Chair, and today, my husband, Steve, serves as treasurer of Lamaze International. I have also enjoyed being a member of ICEA and attending their conferences for many years.

Today, my business partner, Jeanne, and I run the The Family Way, publishing childbirth education materials and training new childbirth educators. I enjoy speaking at conferences around the world. But my greatest joy is my family. As the mother of two boys, I will always be the "mother-in-law." Before my daughter-in-law became pregnant with our first grandchild, I gave her the book, *Pushed,* to read. After she finished it, she called to ask how she could have the birth that she wanted. When she did become pregnant, I was delighted that she chose a combined midwifery-OB practice and invited me to be her doula at both her births. To watch and help her and my son experience the joy and the challenge of natural births were high points of my life. And the end result – everything they say about being a grandparent is true.

Spending time with Ben and his partner, James, and with Brian, Jordan, and our two grandsons are our greatest joys. We also love traveling, rooting for the University of Texas and Rice, and reading. Life is good.

Jeanne Green: I spent my school years in Tulsa, Oklahoma, before moving to San Antonio, Texas, to attend Trinity University. I completed a degree in biology and became a registered medical technologist there. Then I took off to work my way around the world, spending a year of that time in Australia. It was there that I first saw a baby born in a small outback hospital. It was an awesome experience and it touched my heart! A few years later in California my husband and I experienced the birth of our first daughter, and life changed. I didn't realize just how much this birth would affect my life until we moved with our baby from California to Arkansas. The birth culture in those two states was quite different in the early 1970s. In Arkansas there were no childbirth classes, and most mothers were put to sleep for birth. I felt so strongly about the joy I had experienced, being awake and aware of my daughter's birth, that I set about to find like-minded women who joined me on my journey to bring childbirth education to families in Arkansas. We became certified by what is now Lamaze International. A year later, "prepared" fathers were allowed to be present for the birth of their baby. During that time I had two more babies the way I wanted to do it! We moved on to Texas and I joined with new friends to start a childbirth group called *The Family Way*… and I was soon once again "in the family way" with baby number four.

I am a Lamaze Certified Childbirth Educator (LCCE) and a Fellow in the Academy of Certified Childbirth Educators. I have been an active member of Lamaze International, the International Childbirth Education Association, and DONA International. I enjoyed working with Lamaze and InJoy as script writer and class instructor in the DVD, *Celebrate Birth!* I teach classes and seminars, train childbirth educators and doulas, and I love to attend births.

I am thrilled that I have been invited to the births of my eight grandchildren (one set of twins) in the past six years! Earning the title of "Nana" is my greatest accomplishment. Our children, Elaine, David, Whitney, and Emily, and their loved ones and children bring us amazing joy. Gordon and I have traveled the world for career and for pleasure. Being with family, attending births, playing with babies, writing books, teaching, practicing yoga, traveling – life just doesn't get much better than that!

Contents

Breastfeeding

Postpartum and Family

Birth Stories

Workbook

Pregnancy

Pregnancy is your time…a transition stage that enables you to grow into parenthood…. You have nine months in which to slowly grow, evolve, nourish, sustain, and ultimately give birth to a new life.

Sylvia Klein Olkin

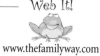

Communicate, Communicate, Communicate

Talking to each other is an important part of any good relationship. And listening is as important as talking. Different personality types, and different sexes, may communicate differently – and so may pregnant women!

For most, pregnancy is a time of good health, good feelings, pride, and fulfillment. But mixed with these good feelings may be fears, aches and pains, mood swings, worries about finances and new responsibilities, and even concerns about leaving behind a "carefree" life-style. Sometimes the father-to-be feels left out, due to all the attention focused on mom. Either or both of you may have mixed feelings about mom's "new body." Because of this, in addition to hormone fluctuations and fatigue, there will be both ups and downs in sexual desires. If these changes aren't talked about openly, misunderstandings, anger, and guilt can result.

When a woman is pregnant she learns a role in life that may be new to her – that of protector and nurturer for her growing baby. She may feel conflict between her need to relax and let go as her body changes, and her need to keep up her pace and image in the work-force. As she tries to do it all, her frustrations and mood swings may become more exaggerated than ever. She needs to talk, to express her feelings, and to be reassured that she is competent and lovable. It may be difficult for her to ask for help. She may not understand her own mood swings, but she wants her partner to understand them. She needs him to be there for her – not to solve her problems, but to listen to her as she unloads her joys and frustrations of pregnancy and her fears and anxieties of birth and parenthood.

When two people are on the same wavelength, thoughts or even words might escape your lips at the same moment. It is as though you are so connected that you hardly need to speak. At other times, you are so misunderstood you may as well be speaking different languages.

Women often think while they talk, but many men use silence and withdrawal to think. As much as she wants him to listen to her express her feelings, and for him to express his, he may want her to allow him to be silent. Don't mistake silence for rejection!

It is important to have patience with one another. Both of you should try to understand one another's needs. If one person does all the giving, the relationship suffers. Riding the waves of the emotions of pregnancy and birth is not easy. Make time to talk and to listen to each other. This helps you form a special closeness and appreciation for one another and a strong base for your new roles as parents.

Talking	Listening
🍃 Some people prefer to focus on only one thing at a time. When you need help with something or just want to talk, give your partner time to change direction.	🍃 Listen to your partner's stories of the day; ask for more detail even when you think there can be no more!
🍃 Tell each other what you need. Don't expect your partner to read your mind.	🍃 Your physical presence, listening ears, and loving arms offer the best solution for many problems.
🍃 Let your partner know when you need time to be heard. "Schedule" it in your busy day.	🍃 Listening to silence may help relieve stress. Quiet time alone with a book or TV is more necessary for some than for others. Honor that time.
🍃 Compliment your partner. Express your love and appreciation for what he or she does for you.	🍃 Support each other in this pregnancy; if you don't know what the other needs, ask.

What's Going On During Pregnancy

	Development of the Baby	Possible Feelings of the Mother	Possible Feelings of the Father
1st Trimester – Adjustment	**By the End of the First Month** Minus 14 days – last menstrual period Day 1 – fertilization Day 6 – implantation Day 14 – missed menstrual period ¼ to ½ inch long All organs present Day 18 – heart beating One month – arm and leg buds **By the End of the Second Month** Human facial features All major body systems laid down Particularly sensitive to chemicals Fetal heart tones may be heard Capable of motion Arms, hands, fingers, legs, feet, toes formed Real bone begins replacing cartilage Milk-tooth buds formed **By the End of the Third Month** Sex can be distinguished Less susceptible to outside forces Fetus kicking, making faces Fetus swallowing, breathing movements	**Physical** Hormonal upheaval Urinary frequency Fatigue Morning sickness Backache **Emotional** Excitement Apprehension Mood swings Cries for anger or joy	**Physical** "Couvade" – may experience physical symptoms similar to mom **Emotional** New sense of responsibility Concerned with mother's mood swings
		Both Mother and Father Pride Often ambivalence precedes acceptance of pregnancy Concern over mother's changing body Sometimes ambivalent to sex	
2nd Trimester – Acceptance	**By the End of the Fourth Month** Fetus recognizable as a human baby Length: 8 to 10 inches Weight: 6 ounces **By the End of the Fifth Month** Quickening – mother feels movement Length: 10-12 inches Weight: ~ 1 pound Hair on head; lanugo (fine hair) on body Capable of hearing Nails on fingers and toes Fetal heart tones (FHT) clearly heard **By the End of the Sixth Month** Possible chance of survival if born now Length: 14 inches Weight: 1¾ pounds Vernix caseosa produced Permanent tooth buds formed Strong grip	**Physical** Hormones in better balance More energy Quickening – feels baby move **Emotional** Less moodiness Feelings of good health and well-being	**Physical** Hears heart tones Feels baby move **Emotional** Gets more emotionally involved Becomes more protective of mother
		Both Mother and Father Sex more appealing Fear of injury to baby Worry over partner	
3rd Trimester – Anticipation	**By the End of the Seventh Month** Weight: 3 pounds Gaining immunities from mother Shedding lanugo **By the End of the Eighth Month** Weight: 5 pounds Probably head down position Gaining immunities from mother **By the End of the Ninth Month** Length: 20 inches Weight: 7 to 7½ pounds Lightening – baby "drops" Gaining immunities from mother	**Physical** Discomforts due to enlarging body Fatigue May not have much interest in sex **Emotional** Body image – feels "glowing" and/or unattractive Nightmares	**Physical** Sees baby move **Emotional** May feel left out Financial worries Concerns over sexual relationship
		Both Mother and Father Excitement about birth mixed with fears for well-being of mother and baby Apprehension about birth experience Concern about parenthood and loss of freedom	

Try This for Comfort

Discomfort	Solution
Nausea	Eat 4 to 5 small meals a day, rather than 3 large meals. Don't let stomach become empty. Eat crackers before arising. Chew crystallized ginger; drink ginger tea; eat salty with sour. Wear motion sickness bands. Eat well balanced diet – especially B vitamins.
Fatigue	Listen to your body – Rest!
Stuffy nose	Try saline nose drops. Use warm compresses.
Backache	Maintain proper posture; use good body mechanics. Wear an abdominal support garment. Try pelvic tilt exercises (page 16).
Constipation	Eat lots of foods with bulk – whole grains, bran, raw vegetables, fresh and dried fruits. Drink lots of water and fruit juices. Establish a daily habit. Get regular exercise such as walking.
Leg cramp	Partner can place the heel of mom's foot in his palm, then gently use his forearm to push the ball of her foot towards her body. Adjust calcium/phosphorus ratio – talk to doctor or midwife. Help prevent with calf stretches (page 17).
Heartburn	Eat small frequent meals; drink more liquids between meals, rather than with meals. Avoid fatty and highly spiced foods. Avoid lying down immediately after a meal. Avoid ice cold, very hot, or carbonated beverages. Talk to your doctor or midwife about using antacids.
Shortness of breath	Maintain correct posture. Slow down. Sleep propped up with pillows.
Swelling in legs and feet	Sit, swim, or walk in water; end shower with cool water. Increase fluids. Sit instead of stand; lie down instead of sit; elevate feet several times a day. Do foot twirls, ankle circles. Eat fewer carbs at dinner; they hold more water than fat and proteins. Apply support hose after legs have been elevated.
Varicose veins	Elevate legs at right angle to body 2 to 5 minutes several times a day. Wear support hose. Try warm bath to soothe legs. Avoid "knees-locked" and legs-crossed positions.
Hemorrhoids	Avoid constipation; increase fiber and water intake. Kegel for circulation (page 18). Apply witch hazel compresses.

Some Helpful Terms

Amniotic sac or "bag of waters." The thin membrane around the baby and the amniotic fluid. At full term, there is about a quart of amniotic fluid in the sac. About ⅓ of this fluid is replaced every hour.

Braxton-Hicks contractions. Usually painless uterine contractions present from the earliest days of pregnancy. The mother may feel them from about the fifth month on. They may occur more often and become stronger as the mother gets closer to the start of true labor.

Contractions. The rhythmic tightening and relaxation of the uterus. They cause the cervix to thin (efface) and open (dilate) and they push the baby out of the uterus. True labor contractions usually come in a regular pattern, gradually get closer together, and gradually increase in intensity. The frequency of the contractions is measured from the beginning of one contraction to the beginning of the next contraction; the duration refers to the length of one contraction; and the intensity refers to the strength of the contraction.

Cervix. The lowest part of the uterus which resembles a "neck" until birth, when it opens into the birth canal (vagina) to allow the baby to pass through.

Dilation (dilatation). The opening up of the cervix so that the baby can pass from the uterus to the birth canal. Measured in centimeters from 0 to 10.

Doula. A professional labor support person or postpartum helper. (See page 31.)

Effacement. The thinning and shortening of the cervix; measured in percentages from 0 to 100.

Endorphins. The body's own pain control. Morphine-like pain inhibitors are produced by the brain in high levels during an unmedicated labor and birth.

Engagement. The entrance of the baby's presenting part into the upper oval of the mother's pelvis. In primigravidas, engagement often takes place about two weeks before the baby's birth. In multigravidas, it can occur as late as the onset of labor.

Episiotomy. A small surgical incision of the perineum made to enlarge the vaginal opening. If one is necessary, it is done just before the birth of the baby.

Fundus. The top or uppermost portion of the uterus.

Lightening. The sensation the mother feels when the baby "drops" down or gradually settles into the pelvis as the presenting part becomes engaged.

Multigravida. A woman pregnant with her second or subsequent child.

Multipara (multip). A woman who has given birth to more than one child.

Perineum. The external tissues surrounding the urethra, vagina, and anus; the space between the vagina and anus where an episiotomy would be done if needed.

Presentation. Refers to the part of the baby which can first be felt through the cervix upon vaginal exam; the part of the baby which will first enter the birth canal:

- *Cephalic.* Head first – occurs in more than 95% of births. May be anterior, posterior, or transverse position.

- *Breech.* One or both feet or buttocks first – occurs in 3.5% of births.

- *Shoulder (transverse lie).* Baby lying sideways in the uterus – occurs in less than 1.5% of births.

Primigravida. A woman pregnant with her first child.

Primipara (primip). A woman who has given birth to her first child.

Station. The relationship of the baby's presenting part to the mother's ischial spines (part of the pelvis). A minus-five station refers to a baby whose presenting part has not yet entered the pelvis or is floating; a zero station refers to a baby whose presenting part is engaged; and a plus-five station refers to a baby whose presenting part is at the perineal floor and birth is about to occur.

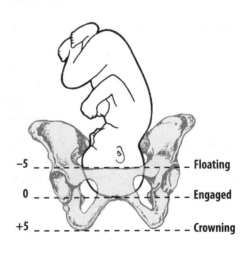

Anatomy of Pregnancy

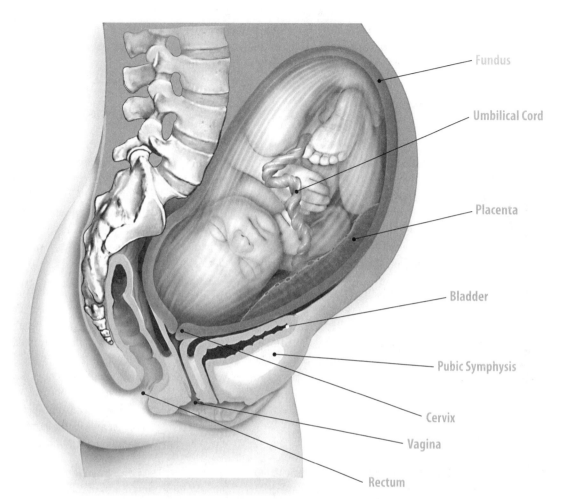

- Fundus
- Umbilical Cord
- Placenta
- Bladder
- Pubic Symphysis
- Cervix
- Vagina
- Rectum

Web It!

Positions and Presentations of the Baby

Cephalic Presentations

Breech Presentation

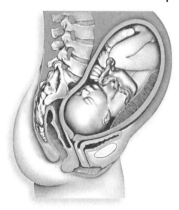

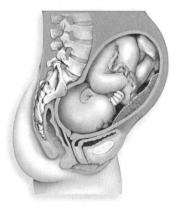

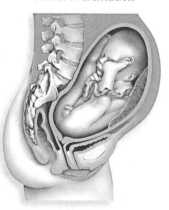

Anterior Position
(Baby's face is facing mom's spine)

The most common position for the baby to be born

Posterior Position
(Back of baby's head is against mom's spine)

"Sunnyside-up"

Frank Breech
(Buttocks first, legs extended)

Most common breech position

Precautions

Pregnancy and breastfeeding are healthy, normal processes for most women. However, during pregnancy and breastfeeding, the developing baby is exposed to toxins that pass to the baby through the mother. For this reason, pregnant and nursing women have questions about what is and what may not be safe. Below are some guidelines for common substances. Your health care provider can give you more information.

	Pregnancy	Breastfeeding
Alcohol	No safe amount of alcohol has been determined for pregnancy. Major health organizations in the U.S. and Canada recommend that pregnant women abstain completely from alcoholic beverages. Heavy drinking, especially in the early months of pregnancy, is associated with Fetal Alcohol Syndrome. This can cause mental retardation, facial malformations, growth retardation, and liver and kidney problems.	According to the American Academy of Pediatrics Committee on Drugs, an occasional drink or light drinking (one or fewer drinks per day) have not been found to be harmful to the nursing baby. However, alcohol is passed freely into breastmilk, and studies have shown that nursing mothers who abuse alcohol may have babies who fail to grow and develop normally
Tobacco	If mother smokes, the baby in the uterus gets less oxygen. This will harm the growth of the baby. Cigarette smoking has been linked to 20 to 30 percent of all low birth-weight babies in the United States. Low birth-weight is the second leading cause of infant deaths in this country.	According to La Leche League, for the mother who smokes twenty or fewer cigarettes per day, the benefits of breastfeeding outweigh the small health risks of passing nicotine to the baby in the breastmilk. However, the more cigarettes the mother smokes, the greater the risks to the baby. For the nursing mother who doesn't quit smoking, it is recommended that she smoke only immediately after nursing her baby. This lowers the amount of nicotine in her milk for the next feeding. Also, the baby should not be around any tobacco smoke.
Caffeine	Studies don't agree on how much caffeine is safe in pregnancy. The American Dietetic Association recommends pregnant women have less than 300 mg of caffeine per day. A "cup of coffee" varies in the amount of caffeine it contains. A "tall" 12 oz. cup of coffee may contain as much as 240 mg of caffeine. Most caffeine-containing teas and sodas contain half as much caffeine as coffee, but some energy drinks contain more. Choose a latte to reduce caffeine and add the benefit of milk!	According to La Leche League, the amount of caffeine in 5 (5 ounce) cups or less of coffee does not cause problems for most breastfeeding mothers and their babies. More caffeine may cause overstimulation of the baby.
Legal Drugs	The safety of prescription drugs as well as many over-the-counter medications may depend on the stage of pregnancy and/or other substances or medications the woman may be taking. Pregnant and breastfeeding women should ask their health care provider before taking any medication.	
Illegal Drugs	Illegal drugs including heroin, marijuana, and cocaine may have devastating effects on the developing baby before birth. Pregnant women should avoid all "street" drugs and seek treatment if they have addictions.	According to the American Academy of Pediatrics, women who use heroin, marijuana, or cocaine should be discouraged from breastfeeding because of the potential dangerous effects of these drugs, which are passed in breastmilk. However, women who are taking 20 mg. or less of methadone to combat heroin addiction can and should breastfeed their babies.

Nutrition

There is no more important issue in pregnancy than nutrition. The unborn baby's growth depends upon what mom eats and drinks. The baby wins if mom eats healthy foods. If her diet is poor, or if she takes in harmful drugs or toxic foods, then the baby is the one to be harmed. Eating a healthy diet is one of the most important things you can do to have a healthy baby. Check your eating habits on various days by using the Diet Evaluation on page 103.

Weight Gain and Exercise

How tall you are and how much you weigh before becoming pregnant determines how much weight you should gain during pregnancy. Women who are underweight before becoming pregnant are encouraged to gain 28 to 40 pounds during pregnancy; normal weight women should gain 25 to 35 pounds; over-weight women should gain 15 to 25 pounds; and obese women should limit their gain to 11 to 20 pounds. Most of your weight gain should take place in the last two trimesters. It is okay if you gain only one to four pounds in the first trimester. If you are carrying multiples, you should take in more calories and gain more weight according to the number of babies. Your health care provider may have special recommendations for you, based on your medical history and life-style. Exercise is considered an important part of a healthy life-style. Healthy pregnant women are encouraged to exercise at least 30 minutes, most, if not all days of the week.

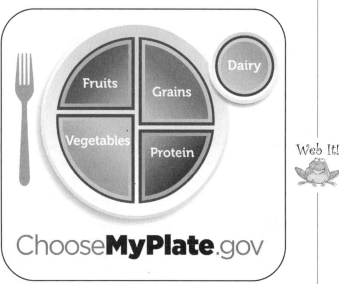

Web It!

Canadian readers can view the Canadian nutrition guide at www.hc-sc.gc.ca/fn-an/nutrition/prenatal/index-eng.php

How Much to Eat

The *Dietary Guidelines for Americans, 2010* stresses eating an amount of food based on your age, health, activity level, and trimester of pregnancy. For example, a healthy 25-year old woman pregnant with one baby who exercises 30 to 60 minutes most days of the week needs no additional calories or food servings in the first trimester of pregnancy. An additional 200 calories are recommended for the second trimester and an additional 400 calories are recommended for the third trimester. An extra serving from the Dairy Group and from Protein Foods Group can easily provide extra calories. Serving sizes for all the food groups for this woman are indicated on the following two pages.

Visit this website: <www.choosemyplate.gov> then click on "Pregnant and Breastfeeding." Enter your own information as requested to determine the number of calories and servings from each food group recommended for you during each trimester.

Balance, Variety, and Moderation

The MyPlate icon shows that half of your plate should be fruits and vegetables and half should be grains and protein. Add the circle of dairy products to meet your calcium needs. If your plate doesn't look like this at every meal, try to make up for it by the end of a day to get a balanced diet.

A variety of protein foods may be baked, broiled, boiled, or grilled. Choose lean meats, and add more fish, beans, peas, nuts, and seeds to your diet. Tofu (soy bean curd) and tempeh are good vegetarian sources of protein.

Eat at least 3 ounces of whole grain bread, cereal, crackers, rice, or pasta every day. Choose a variety of whole grains such at quinoa, buckwheat, rolled oats, whole barley, and whole couscous.

Eat more dark green and orange vegetables. Dry beans and peas count as veggies or proteins.

If you don't or can't consume milk, choose lactose-free products or other calcium sources. Soy milk is fortified with calcium and vitamins A and D, so is considered part of the Dairy Group.

Choose fresh, frozen, canned, or dried fruit. Juice drinks are just "empty calories" of sugar. Drink 100% fruit juice.

Be aware of the amount of "empty calories" in solid fats and added sugars that you eat and drink. Moderation is the key. A few sweets aren't harmful to you and your baby, but a low-nutrient diet is.

Healthy Food Choices

Grains
7 to 9 ounces daily
Note: Many portions often considered "normal" are actually several servings. For instance, a large bagel is 4 ounces!

Many of these choices are high in complex carbohydrates; vitamins such as B vitamins (including folate) and vitamin E; minerals; and fiber. Eat products from a variety of grains such as wheat, oats, rice, and corn. Choose whole-grain foods rather than processed or fortified foods. When reading labels, look for *whole-wheat* as the first ingredient for breads, crackers, pasta, and cereals, rather than *wheat flour*. Not all brown bread contains whole-wheat and not all whole-grain crackers are brown. Look at the label rather than the color. "Make half your grains whole."

Vegetables
3 to 3 ½ cups daily

Vegetables provide carbohydrates; vitamins such as vitamin A, vitamin C, and folate; minerals such as iron and magnesium; and valuable fiber. They are naturally low in fat and calories. To insure that you meet your needs for the various vitamins, it is important to choose from a variety of vegetables. Eat deep yellow and dark green leafy vegetables often. To obtain the most vitamins, choose vegetables in this order: fresh, frozen, canned.

Fruits
2 cups daily

Fruits also provide carbohydrates; vitamins such as vitamin A, vitamin C, and folate; minerals such as potassium; and valuable fiber. Although 100% fruit juices are healthy beverages, you will get additional vitamins and fiber by eating the whole fruit. Choose citrus fruits, melons, and berries regularly to make sure you are getting enough vitamin C.

Dairy
3 cups daily

Dairy products provide protein, vitamins A and D, and minerals such as calcium and phosphorus. Serving sizes for dairy products are determined by calcium content. Because cottage cheese is lower in calcium than most other cheeses, one cup of cottage cheese counts as only ½ serving of the Dairy Group. On the other hand, ricotta cheese is much higher in calcium, so that only ½ cup counts as one serving of the Dairy Group. If you have trouble digesting milk, you may need nutritional counseling to insure that you get all the nutrients you need from this food group.

Protein Foods
6 to 6 ½ ounces daily

The recommended intake for protein during pregnancy is 60 grams per day. Some protein choices are excellent sources of protein *(chicken breast, 3½ oz. = 29 grams; tuna, 3 oz. = 23 grams)* while other choices are poorer sources *(bacon, 2 slices = 4 grams; fast-food fish sandwich = 14 grams)*. Complete proteins are needed for growth and development of the baby. Animal sources (meat, milk, and eggs) provide complete proteins, while plant sources (grains, dried beans, seeds, and nuts) are incomplete proteins. You must combine incomplete proteins from different sources to make complete proteins. If you are a vegetarian, you may need nutritional counseling to make sure you are getting all the nutrients you need.

Oils
6 to 8 teaspoons daily
(Note: 3 teaspoons = 1 tablespoon)

We do need some fat in our diet in order to metabolize foods properly and absorb certain vitamins. However, it is easy to get too many fats and the wrong kinds of fats in our diet. For salad oils, spreads, and cooking oils use olive oil or canola oil as first choice, vegetable oils (corn, safflower, sunflower) as second choice. Least preferred are saturated fats such as palm oil and fats from animal sources. Because most processed sweets add only empty calories and/or fats to your diet, fruits are better choices for desserts and snacks.

Supplements

According to *Nutrition During Pregnancy,* released by the National Academy of Sciences, normal, healthy pregnant women should be able to obtain most needed nutrients from diet alone. The only supplements that healthy, pregnant women may need are iron and folic acid. The American College of Obstetricians and Gynecologists (ACOG) does NOT recommend restriction of salt during pregnancy.

Water

Pregnant women have up to 40% more blood volume by the time they reach term. To support this increase in blood volume, pregnant women need extra fluids. Milk, fruit juices, and water are the recommended beverages. Drink to thirst and stay well-hydrated.

Equal to a 1 ounce serving:
1 slice of bread, small muffin, small roll
½ mini-bagel or ½ English muffin
1 small flour tortilla or 1 corn tortilla
½ cup cooked cereal, pasta, or rice
1 cup processed cereal (read package)
3 cups of popcorn, popped

100% whole-wheat products have more B vitamins and fiber than either brown or white wheat flour bread or crackers. Corn tortillas contain less fat and fewer calories than flour tortillas. Baked corn chips have much less fat than fried chips. Make pancakes or waffles from whole-grain flour, or add wheat bran to the batter. Oatmeal and shredded wheat are two high-nutrition cereals. Cheese melted on mini shredded wheat squares, air popped popcorn, and rye or whole-grain crackers make good snacks.

Equal to 1 cup vegetables:
1 cup cooked vegetables
2 cups raw leafy greens
1 cup vegetable juice
1 medium potato (2 ½ to 3 inch diameter)
1 cup cooked dry beans or peas

Salsa and pico de gallo may be enjoyed with a meal or as a snack to add vitamins A and C. Leafy greens (the darker, the better) such as spinach, broccoli, Brussels sprouts, and lettuces are high in vitamins A and C and folate. Tomatoes and green and red peppers used in salads or sauces are good sources of vitamin C. Make your plate as colorful as possible and you will more easily get the nutrients you need.

Equal to 1 cup fruit:
1 cup 100% fruit juice
½ cup dried fruit
1 small apple; 1 small banana; 1 medium pear

Fruits make excellent snacks and desserts. Choose fresh fruits; 100% fruit juices; and frozen, canned (in its own juice), or dried fruits. Avoid fruits canned in heavy syrup unless you are trying to add extra calories to your diet.

Equal to 1 cup milk:
1 cup milk
1 cup yogurt
½ cup some soft cheeses such as ricotta
1½ ounces of hard cheese such as cheddar
2 ounces processed cheese
1 cup frozen yogurt or pudding made with milk

Calcium quantities are not affected by fat content, so whenever possible choose the nonfat or lowfat item for heart-healthy eating. Even most frozen desserts are available in lowfat or nonfat varieties. Two-percent milk is not low-fat; it must be 1% or less to meet low-fat guidelines. If you are trying to increase weight gain, try the harder cheeses and whole milk products.

Equal to 1 ounce protein foods:
1 ounce cooked lean meat, poultry, or fish
1 egg
¼ cup cooked beans or peas; ½ cup bean soup
1 tablespoon nut butter
2 tablespoons hummus
½ ounce (⅛ cup) nuts or seeds
¼ cup tofu (soybean curd)

Complete proteins (animal sources): For heart-healthy eating, chicken, turkey, fish, liver, lean pork, and lean beef are all good sources. Egg whites or egg substitutes may be used in cooking, for breakfast, or in salads. *Incomplete proteins (plant sources):* Some popular ways to combine incomplete proteins to make complete proteins include: cereal with milk, macaroni with cheese, red beans with rice, split pea soup with whole-grain crackers, and peanut butter on whole-wheat bread. Dry beans and peas may be counted in either the Vegetables or Protein Foods Groups.

1 tablespoon (1 pat) butter = 14 grams of fat
1 tablespoon mayonnaise = 12 grams of fat
1 cup of 2% milk = 5 grams of fat
1 cup of 1% milk = 2 ½ grams of fat
1 ounce of hard cheese = 8 grams of fat
1 egg = 6 grams of fat
3 ounces skinless chicken = 4 grams of fat
3 ounces lean sirloin beef = 7 grams of fat

Read food labels carefully and aim for no more than 30% of your daily calories from fat. To determine the number of calories from fat in a food, multiply the number of grams of fat by 9. To determine the percentage of calories from fat in a food, divide the number of calories from fat by the total number of calories in the food. The fats in meat, poultry, and eggs are considered solid fats, while the fats in seafood, nuts, and seeds are considered oils.

Do you know? . . .

Good nutrition in pregnancy is linked with

- healthier babies,
- more energy (less fatigue),
- better pattern of weight gain (and weight loss postpartum),
- less premature labor,
- greater elasticity of tissues (less need for episiotomy), and
- more rapid healing after birth.

Food FAQs

Why is folic acid so important for pregnant women? Is there a difference between folic acid and folate? How much should I take?

Fewer babies have been born with neural tube defects (birth defects of the brain and spinal cord) in the US and Canada since folic acid fortification of foods was started in the late 1990s. Folic acid is the synthetic form of Vitamin B-9 that is in fortified products and in supplements. Folate is the natural vitamin in whole foods. They have the same effects.

Pregnant women are advised to take in 600 mcg of folate equivalents from all sources every day (400 mcg of folic acid in addition to food forms of folate). Sources of food folate include beans and peas, oranges, and dark-green leafy vegetables such as spinach and kale. (Think of foliage = leaf = folate.)

Are garbanzo beans (chickpeas) that are used to make humus considered a vegetable or a protein food?

Dry beans and peas are considered both as a vegetable and as a protein food. You may count them in either group when you total your daily or weekly portions.

Are green beans and snow peas considered protein foods like pinto beans and black-eyed peas?

No, the green pea, snow pea, or English pea is significantly lower in protein content than dry beans and peas (such as black-eyed peas, navy beans, and kidney beans) and so are listed with starchy vegetables and not with Protein Foods. Green (string) beans are grouped with other vegetables such as onions, lettuce, celery, and cabbage because their nutrient content is similar to those foods.

Many plants differ in their nutrient content based on their stage of maturity at harvest, and green peas vs. split peas are a good example of this. Fresh, frozen, or canned green peas have about half the protein content per cup than dry split peas, and a much lower calorie level.

What can I do to add whole-grains to my diet if I don't like to eat whole-wheat bread? Are enriched breads a good substitute?

Try buckwheat pancakes, barley soup, tabouli, popcorn, or oatmeal muffins for a change. You might like breads that combine whole grains and refined grains. But be aware that words like "multigrain," "3-grain," or even "10-grain," don't guarantee that the bread actually contains any whole grains. Some examples of whole-grain ingredients include buckwheat, bulgur, millet, oatmeal, quinoa, rolled oats, brown or wild rice, whole-grain barley, whole rye, and whole wheat. Here is a quick and easy breakfast in a mug:

> *Stir together in a large coffee mug:*
> *⅓ cup oatmeal, ½ teaspoon baking powder, 1 large egg, dash of salt.*
> *Optional: add 1 teaspoon sugar, dash of cinnamon, or some mashed banana or berries.*
> *Microwave for one minute and dump out of mug. Cut in half and add butter or cream cheese.*

"Refined" grains that are processed to give them a finer texture and a longer shelf-life lose dietary fiber, iron, and many B vitamins in the processing of the grain. "Enriched" grain products are refined grains that have B vitamins and iron added back to them. They are also often high in solid fats and sugars. The recommendation is that you make half the grains you eat, whole grains.

Is it true that I shouldn't eat any soft cheeses, sushi, and deli meats while I'm pregnant?

Not exactly. Milk products and soft cheeses that are not pasteurized shouldn't be eaten in pregnancy, but you can find brie, blue, and feta cheeses that have been pasteurized, which you may enjoy. The heat process in pasteurization kills the bacteria that are unsafe for unborn babies. In the same way, undercooked or raw meat, fish, shellfish, or eggs as well as raw sprouts could cause a problem. (It takes heat to kill bacteria and parasites that could harm the baby.) Avoid sushi made with raw fish or with fish having high levels of mercury. Reheat deli meats to steaming hot. All fresh fruits and vegetables should be washed thoroughly before eating.

How can I get enough iron in my diet so that I won't become anemic? Is it necessary to take an iron supplement?

It's difficult to get enough iron in food sources alone, even for a very health-conscious eater! Choose foods that supply heme iron such as lean meat and poultry and seafood. Heme iron is used more easily by your body than the non-heme iron that is in plant foods such as white beans, lentils, and spinach. Do eat both forms. Vitamin C-rich foods help your body to absorb more of the iron that you take in, but tea can decrease your absorption of non-heme iron taken at the same meal. So eating orange segments with a spinach salad or drinking orange juice to take an iron tablet will increase the iron you absorb. But drinking tea with non-heme iron sources will decrease your absorption of the iron at that meal. Women who are pregnant are advised to take an iron supplement as recommended by an obstetrician or other health care provider.

Do all fish contain mercury that could harm my baby? If shrimp and tuna are the only kinds of seafood I like, will that be enough to eat?

Pregnant and nursing women should eat a variety of small fish, rather than large fish. Larger fish such as tilefish, shark, swordfish, and king mackerel are older, so may accumulate high levels of mercury. Women who are pregnant or breastfeeding can eat all types of tuna, including white (albacore) and light canned tuna, but should limit white tuna and fresh tuna steaks to 6 ounces per week because they are higher in methyl mercury.

Because fish contain valuable nutrients necessary for the baby's brain and eye development, it is recommended that pregnant and breastfeeding women eat at least 8 and up to 12 ounces of a variety of seafood that are low in mercury each week. This should be about 20 % of your protein foods. Seafood includes fish, such as salmon, tuna, trout, and tilapia, and shellfish, such as shrimp, crab, and oysters. If you do not eat this much seafood, ask your health care provider about taking fish oil supplements to help you get enough Omega-3 fatty acids.

How can I make myself eat more fruits and vegetables when it is easier to eat meat and potatoes on the go?

Don't leave your house without a piece of fruit, raw veggies, or a 100% fruit or vegetable juice or smoothie to drink. Eating snacks in mid-morning and mid-afternoon is important in pregnancy. Keep them handy on eye-level in your refrigerator to grab when you come home from work or during your day at home. Add a salad or lots of veggies (avocado, mushrooms, peppers, cucumbers, etc.) on a sandwich for a fast-food lunch. Vegetables are easy to add to any dinner at home. Steam fresh spinach, corn, squash, or peas in just minutes in the microwave, steamer, or stove-top. Stir-fry peppers, onions, green beans, or broccoli while the pasta boils. Grill asparagus, mushrooms, zucchini, and onions while the burger cooks. When dining out, add a salad to your meal or request that fruit or veggies be substituted for fried potatoes. Choose fruit for dessert (even if it's berries with ice cream or sherbet!). Vegetables provide folate, potassium, fiber, and vitamins to help grow a healthy baby. There is nothing wrong with potatoes that are baked or boiled, just don't add the fat to fry them! Perhaps knowing that vegetables and fruits may be protective against certain types of cancer and reduce your risk of heart attack and stroke will help to motivate you to form life-long healthy eating habits for you and your children. They will eat what you eat. So, slow down and eat right!

Remember this advice from *ChooseMyPlate.gov:*

- Make at least half your grains whole grains
- Vary your veggies
- Focus on fruit
- Get your calcium rich foods
- Go lean with protein
- Find your balance between food and physical activity
- Keep food safe to eat

Body Mechanics

The way you sit, stand, move, and relax while you are pregnant can affect the way you feel. The weight of the baby pulling forward on the uterus where it attaches to the low back can cause backache. The baby's presence also changes mother's center of gravity. The increased blood volume can cause muscle aches, swelling, and/or decreased feeling in the legs and arms. Hormones that soften ligaments may add to muscle aches. The following suggestions for positions and movement should help you be more comfortable now, in labor, and throughout life.

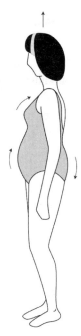

Standing Posture

Stand with feet about 3 inches apart with toes turned slightly outward.

Keep hips tucked under (pelvic tilt).

Keep shoulders back but do not let the back arch.

Keep head back over shoulders.

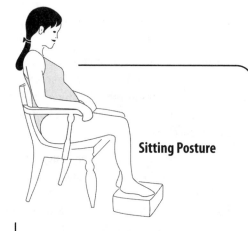

Sitting Posture

Sit in a chair with a firm but comfortable back support, with head over shoulders.

Arm rest should not be too low or too high.

Keep knees slightly higher than hips.

Small pads behind neck and low back may be added for comfort.

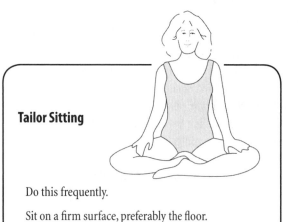

Tailor Sitting

Do this frequently.

Sit on a firm surface, preferably the floor.

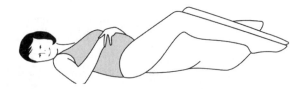

Positioning on Back

Place 2 or 3 pillows under knees.

Place a rolled bath towel under the bend of neck. If using a pillow at the head, also place it well under the shoulders.

Keep arms at sides or resting on stomach.

(Lying on back recommended only before 20 weeks or during postpartum.)

Stooping, Lifting, and Carrying Objects

Place one foot ahead of other before bending at knees.

Straighten legs, keep back straight.

Lift object slightly to one side.

Carry object waist high, close to body.

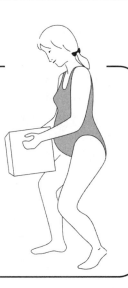

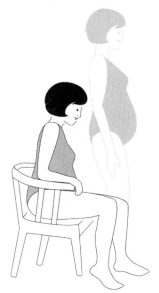

Rising From Low Furniture

Scoot hips forward to edge of chair.

Place one foot slightly forward and rotate hips in the direction of forward foot.

Keep back straight.

Use arms and large thigh muscles to lift yourself up.

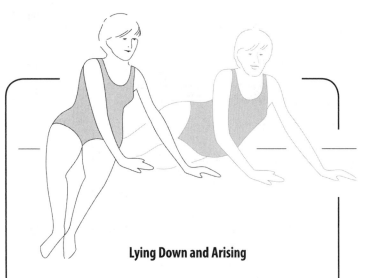

Lying Down and Arising

From sitting position, use hands to walk self down to side-lying.

If rolling to back, turn shoulders and hips as one unit.

Return to side-lying again as one unit.

Pause for a moment before rising.

Side-Lying

Lie on side with knees bent.

Place pillow between knees, under upper arm, under head, and under uterus as needed for comfort.

Lower arm may either be in front under pillow or behind the back.

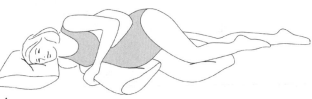

Birth Fitness

Do all exercises slowly without bouncing or jerking. You should feel stretch, but not pain. Start with a small number of repetitions and gradually increase. It does not take long exercise sessions to ease aches, increase flexibility and circulation, and generally make you feel better. These exercises can be done while watching television or during short stretch breaks throughout the day (see page 100).

All pelvic tilt exercises may be done to ease backache during pregnancy and labor. The pelvic tilt on all fours may be helpful in rotating a posterior baby during labor.

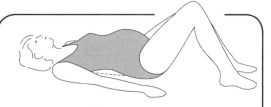

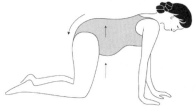

Pelvic Tilt on Back (before 20 weeks)

Lie on back with knees bent.

Tighten the abdominal (abs) muscles, pushing the low back flat against the floor.

Hold for 5 counts; relax; repeat.

Variation:
    While holding the pelvic tilt, bring one knee towards the chest. Grasp the knee with both hands and pull towards the chest until you feel a good stretch (not pain) in the back muscles.
    Hold 30 seconds, then return leg to starting position and repeat with other leg.

Pelvic Tilt on All Fours

Assume all fours position, keeping back straight (do not let lower back sag).

Tighten abs so pelvis tucks under and lower back rounds.

Hold for 5 counts; relax; repeat.

Variation:
    Hold the pelvic tilt while you "swish" hips from side-to-side. Head turns as if ear will touch hips on the same side.

Repeat.

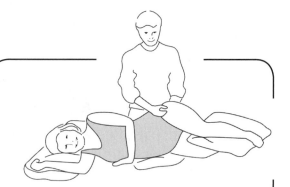

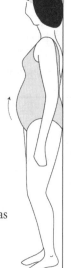

Standing Pelvic Tilt

Stand with knees softened (slightly bent).

Tighten abs and press the small of the back flat, as if against an imaginary wall.

Hold this position for one minute.

Relax.

Repeat often if standing for long periods.

Variation:
    May put hands under belly to lift abdomen as you tilt your pelvis (see page 47).

Passive Pelvic Tilt

Mom lies on her side with knees bent. Partner positions himself behind mom's hips.

Using his hand nearest her head, he places his palm on the top of her hip.

His other hand is placed on her tail bone.

He slowly rotates the top of her hip back toward himself as he puts gentle pressure on the tailbone.

Release – repeat.

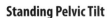

Wall Stretch

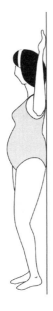

Stand against the wall with knees slightly bent.

Place shoulders, elbows, and wrists against the wall with elbows bent and fingers pointing upwards.

Slowly slide arms up the wall, straightening elbows.

Once arms are overhead, try to pull belly up and in so the back flattens against the wall.

Slide arms back down to the starting position.

Relax abdominals.

Repeat.

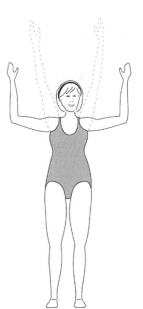

Calf Stretch Against Wall

Stand 2-3 feet back from wall.

Move left foot in towards wall. Pull in belly. Bend left knee, placing hands on wall. Lean in towards wall, keeping head, chest, hips, and right heel in a straight line.

Hold 30-60 seconds while feeling a mild stretch in the right calf.

Change legs and repeat.

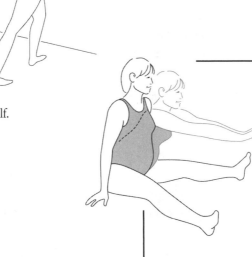

Tailor Stretch

Tilt pelvis and hold it.

Extend legs with knees straight. Extend both arms and reach forward slowly until you feel a mild stretch.

Return to starting position.

Repeat.

Wall Squat

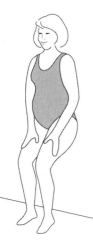

Hold a standing pelvic tilt position with back against a wall.

Slowly slide upper body down the wall until knees are bent as if sitting on a stool.

Hold this position with contracted thighs and abs while relaxing all muscles not being used.

Add:
1. Tighten and release pelvic floor.
2. Use the contracted thighs to simulate uterine contractions while practicing breathing patterns.

Slowly return to standing position.

Kegel Exercises

Many people are not aware of the pelvic floor or pubococcygeus (PC) muscle. Yet the benefits of reaching and keeping good tone in this muscle are many and include:

- Prevention of urinary "dribbling" when coughing or laughing.

- Possible prevention of need for surgery later in life to pull up a "sagging" uterus or other pelvic organs.

- Less discomfort from pelvic exams.

- A shorter and easier second stage of labor (actual birth of the baby).

- Faster healing from episiotomy repair and/or hemorrhoids.

- Greater pleasure during sexual intercourse. Regular exercise every day can strengthen the PC muscle. This has enabled some women to reach orgasm more consistently during intercourse. These exercises done by men can help sustain erections to allow the woman more time to achieve orgasm.

- In men, a possible decrease in likelihood of developing prostate problems by enhancing circulation and support.

The pelvic floor muscle stretches from the pubic symphysis in front to the "tailbone" in back and forms a "sling" of support for the bladder, the uterus, the vagina, and part of the rectum. The muscle fibers surround the opening of the bladder (urethra), the vagina, and the rectum (anus).

To locate this muscle, sit on the toilet with your legs spread apart. Start to urinate, then stop the stream of urine. You should contract the PC muscle when you do this, not the buttocks or abdomen. Hold it tight, then release. Repeat until you learn to control the PC muscle. When you know you are contracting the right muscle, don't start and stop the flow of urine except as an occasional check. Just tighten this muscle after you empty your bladder, or add "Kegels" to any daily routine such as answering the phone, driving a car, standing in line, etc.

To strengthen the PC muscle, try these variations of the Kegel exercise:

Flicks – Contract, then release the PC muscle for one to two seconds (tighten for one-two seconds; release for one-two seconds; repeat). Do these contractions in groups of ten; about ten times each day.

Extended Kegel – Contract the PC muscle and *hold*. Begin by contracting as tightly as you can for 5 seconds and work up to holding for 10 - 20 seconds. The muscle may tire after one extended Kegel, so do these at intervals throughout the day, up to ten times each day. Form a life-long habit of tightening the PC muscle right after you urinate.

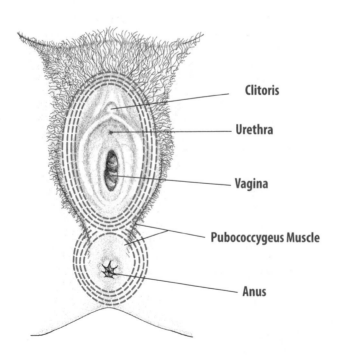

Clitoris

Urethra

Vagina

Pubococcygeus Muscle

Anus

Elevator Exercise – Imagine that your pelvic floor muscle is an elevator. Contract the muscle, slowly tightening it more and more as you go up in the elevator – second, third, fourth, and finally to the fifth floor. Now, slowly release the tension in the pelvic floor going down in the elevator – fourth, third, second, first floor, and basement. The basement is where the muscle should be at the actual moment of birth. Finally, contract back to the first floor level and keep this tone at all times.

Physical therapists who specialize in women's health are good resources for pelvic floor problems as well as for other discomforts of pregnancy.

ACOG Guidelines for Exercise

Web It!

The American College of Obstetricians and Gynecologists (ACOG) recommends a total of 30 minutes or more of moderate exercise on most, if not all, days of the week for pregnant women without medical complications. This may be done all at one time or in shorter sessions. If you haven't been active, start slowly and build up to 30 minutes or more.

Exercise can help you feel better by increasing your energy, relieving or preventing aches and pains of pregnancy, lifting your spirits, improving posture, controlling gestational diabetes, and helping you relax and sleep. The type of exercise you can safely do depends on your health and fitness level. Avoid activities with a high risk of falling or hurting the abdomen such as downhill or water skiing, racquet sports, horseback riding, scuba diving, or contact sports.

Start your workout with stretching and warming up. Move into slow, low-impact activities such as walking, swimming, or cycling. Wear the right shoes with good padding and support for your activities. Wear a sports bra that fits well and gives good support. If you can't talk normally during your workout, you are working too hard. Take a break if you need one. Never exercise until you are exhausted. Drink plenty of fluid before, during, and after your workout. Follow intense exercise with cooling down for 5-10 minutes. Slow your pace little by little and end your workout by gently stretching. Don't stretch too far, though. This can injure the tissue that connects your joints. Reduce your workout levels in late pregnancy. Exercise that may have been easy earlier in pregnancy becomes harder as your belly expands.

Get up slowly after lying or sitting on the floor. Once you're standing, walk in place briefly. Avoid motionless standing and exercising on your back after the first trimester, because your blood circulation could decrease and cut down the blood flow to your baby.

Don't do jerky, bouncy, or high-impact motions. Jumping, jarring motions or quick direction changes can strain your joints and cause pain. Avoid deep knee bends, full sit-ups, double leg lifts, and straight-leg toe touches, which could strain the abdominal and back muscles.

Be sure to discuss any type exercise you'd like to try with your doctor. Here are some options:

- *Walking.* If you were not active before getting pregnant, walking is the ideal way to start an exercise program. Try to walk briskly for 30 minutes most, if not all, days of the week.

- *Swimming.* This is great for your body because it works many different muscles. The water supports your weight so you avoid injury and muscle strain. Stay off the diving board, though. Hitting the water with great force can be harmful.

- *Jogging.* If you were a runner before you became pregnant, you can keep it up now. Be careful, though. Avoid getting too hot. Stop if you have pain or feel too tired. Drink plenty of water to replace the fluid you lose in sweat.

- *Aerobics.* Low-impact aerobics is a safe and good way to keep your heart and lungs strong. There are aerobics classes designed just for pregnant women. Water aerobics also is a good activity. It combines the benefits of swimming and aerobics.

- *Yoga or Pilates.* These programs focus on healthy breathing techniques, stretching and strengthening muscles, and improving flexibility.

Exercise can help prepare your body for labor. It will give you a head start in getting back in shape after your baby is born. A return to physical activity after pregnancy has been associated with decreased incidence of postpartum depression.

Signs of a Problem

If you have any of these symptoms when you exercise, stop your workout and call your caregiver:

- Dizziness or faintness
- Headache
- Increased shortness of breath
- Uneven or rapid heartbeat
- Chest pain
- Trouble walking or calf pain, swelling

- Pain
- Vaginal bleeding
- Uterine contractions that continue after rest
- Fluid gushing or leaking from your vagina
- Decreased fetal movement

Taken from *Your Pregnancy and Birth* by the American College of Obstetricians and Gynecologists (ACOG): Washington, DC, © 2005.

On the Ball!

Benefits of using a "Birth Ball" before, during, and after labor

When you sit on a ball, you use abdominal and lower back muscles to help keep your balance. Your pelvis tilts forward, which may help the baby move into a good position. While sitting on the ball, moving your hips for comfort and balance comes naturally. Rocking your pelvis and shifting weight while upright can increase blood circulation, lessen back pain, and improve posture. The gentle pressure of the ball may help relieve discomfort from hemorrhoids and pressure on the pelvic floor. Rocking or gentle bouncing may comfort your baby before and after birth! Try sitting on a ball at a desk or while watching TV, as well as using one in an exercise program.

> ### "Birth Ball" safety
>
> ❧ Sit on the ball barefooted or wearing rubber soled shoes.
>
> ❧ The ball should fit like a chair.
>
> ❧ Hips, knees, and ankles should each be bent to 90°.
>
> ❧ Be near a support for balance if you need it.

Positions and Movements to Try

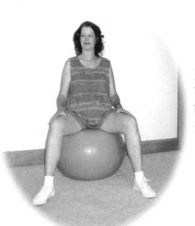

Move in a circular or figure-eight motion while sitting on the ball. This relaxes the back and hips and helps you keep your balance. Add pelvic tilts, moving forward and back, or sway from side-to-side.

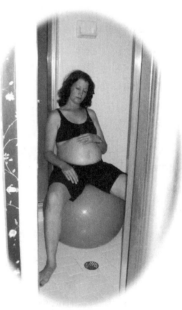

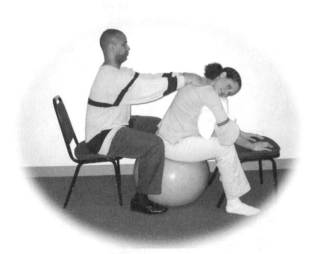

Sit on the ball leaning forward. Release into a pillow on a table, bed, or chair. This helps relieve back pain by moving the baby forward.

The ball may be taken into the shower to sit on while you enjoy the sensations of the warm water.

Kneel on the floor or on the bed with the ball in front of you. Lean over the ball, rolling it forward and back to find a comfortable position for your upper body to rest. Your arms may hug the ball, or be relaxed hanging over it. Your partner may apply back pressure to help relieve pain.

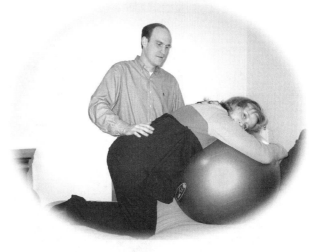

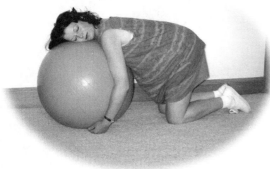

A kneeling position allows for free movement of the pelvis, while gravity encourages the largest and heaviest part of the baby to rotate off mom's back to an anterior position. Putting the weight of the upper body on the ball keeps weight off the wrists.

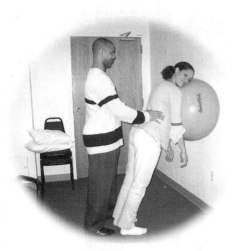

Standing while leaning on a ball that is placed on the wall, a bed, or table, encourages pelvic swaying and rotation, which may help relieve pain and encourage the baby to come down. Standing with your back on the ball against the wall offers pleasant pressure for an aching back, or support for a wall-squat position.

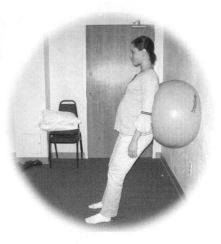

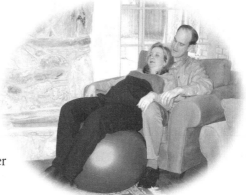

Sitting on the ball, lean back into your partner who is sitting on a chair behind you.

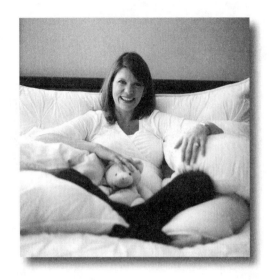

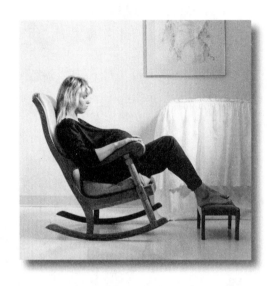

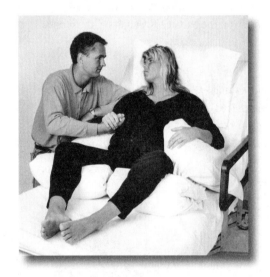

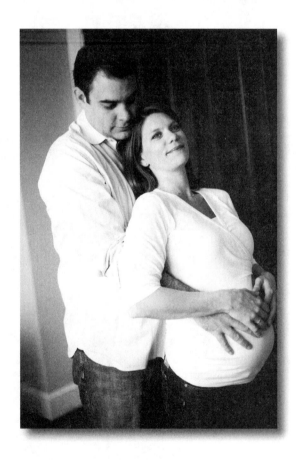

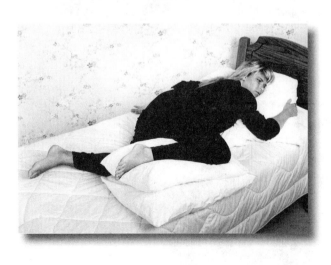

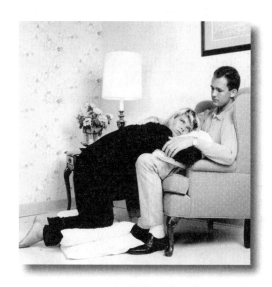

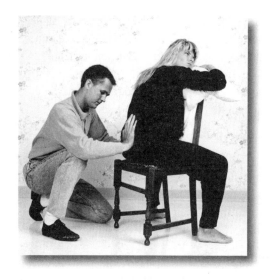

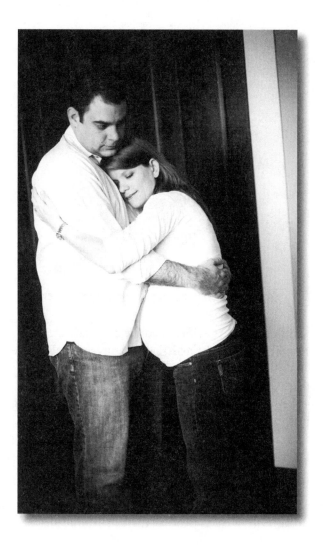

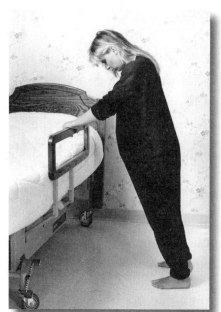

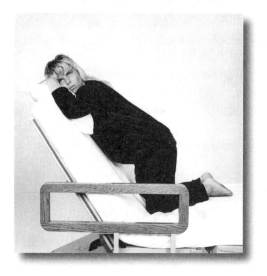

Active Relaxation Techniques

Active relaxation is the ability to "tune in" to your body to release tension in your muscles. It doesn't mean to "tune out" and fall asleep. Relaxing isn't easy for all people, but with practice anyone can learn to let go of tension. Different people respond to different relaxation techniques. Try each of the following techniques, then use what works best for you. Learning to relax is important for labor and birth, but it will also be used in the weeks, months, and years that follow. When any stressful situation arises (dentist visits, freeway driving, baby crying, medical tests, etc.), think *relax*; you will gain control over your body and reduce stress and pain. Become aware of how tense or relaxed you are at different times (see page 99).

Partner's Role

The best way for the partner to help someone else relax is for him to be able to relax himself. Make practice time a team effort; both of you learn to relax, and both learn to check for areas of tension. Talk about what increases relaxation and what causes tension in each of you. The tone of your voice and the firmness of your touch can affect relaxation in your mate. The partner should look for tension, feel for tension, and coax tension away with both verbal cues and touch.

Setting the Stage

While it's both possible and desirable to be able to relax in either chaos or calm, it is easier to learn the techniques when the environment is favorable. During practice sessions (and while you are in labor), think of calming all your senses. Check the following and adjust for comfort:

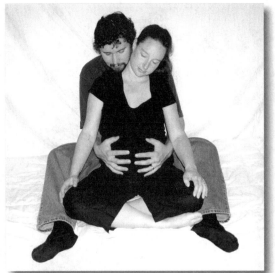

- sight – lighting comfortable; focal point
- sounds – music or silence
- smell – fragrances or fresh air
- taste – water, flavored ice, mouthwash
- touch – temperature (fan, warm or cool packs)
- touch – texture (blanket, pillow, toy)

Get Ready to Relax

- Environment check
- Quick body scan
- Tension release exercises
- Comfortable position
- Focus
- Deep, relaxing, cleansing breath

After you have adjusted your environment, scan your body from head to toe. If you find a tense or painful spot, try to release tension with exercises like head rotations (left, forward, right), shoulder rolls, shaking arms and hands, ankle rolls, and pelvic tilts.

Find a comfortable position with every part of your body supported and joints bent. Use pillows under head, knees, and arms. Relax in sitting, side-lying, and semi-reclining positions. As your ability to relax improves, practice in walking and standing positions too. You will labor in all these positions .

Signal your body to relax by finding a focal point and taking a deep, cleansing breath. Try each of the following active relaxation techniques. Suggested practice sessions may be found on pages 104-106.

Progressive Relaxation

Progressive relaxation is the technique of moving through the body, releasing one muscle group at a time until you have relaxed your entire body. At first it may help to locate tension by either contracting or stretching a muscle group (see Progressive Tense/Release practice exercise on page 104). Practice this exercise until you can simply release by mentally progressing down your body, as in the following scenario.

- Begin by relaxing the muscles of your head and face. Release down the back of your neck, across your shoulders and arms, down your chest, abdomen and back, all the way down your legs to your toes. Breathe slowly, releasing more and more with each exhalation. Each time you release a muscle, concentrate on the positioning of that muscle and on the feeling of complete relaxation.

- It may help to think of a comforting touch smoothing gently from your brow, up into your hair, over the top of your head, and down your body.

Selective Relaxation — *Neuromuscular control*

Selective relaxation consists of contracting one muscle group while keeping all other muscles relaxed. When the uterus contracts during labor, there is a tendency for the other muscles of the body to contract in response to it. Tension travels through the body, sapping energy and increasing pain. Selective relaxation serves as a rehearsal for labor. The muscle you hold tight simulates a uterine contraction as you learn to relax all other muscles. It takes practice to learn this skill, but the benefits will show in labor. It is most helpful for the partner to check for relaxation. Examples:

Contract right arm … *release* all other muscles … *release* right arm

Contract jaws … *relax* the rest of the body … *release* jaws

Contract abdominals and pelvic floor … *release* pelvic floor … *release* abdominals

Contract left arm, right leg … *release* other muscles … *release* right leg, left arm

Autogenic Phrases

Phrases that are repeated over and over can help you relax each part of your body. Think about how relaxation feels to you, then describe those sensations. You may use the same sensation for each muscle group like this:

- my feet are warm,
- my hands are warm,
- my shoulders are warm;

or describe each muscle with a different sensation:

- my hands feel warm,
- my arms are loose,
- my feet are heavy.

You may say the phrases aloud or silently, or you may listen to someone read them. Pause between phrases. Use phrases that are positive for you so that you are refreshed by this exercise. For some pregnant women, the *last* thing they want to feel is warm and heavy! You may add some positive affirmations about your baby and your general state of well-being when you do this exercise: My baby is strong and healthy…. I feel peaceful and calm (see *Relaxing Words* on page 105).

Visual Imagery

Visual imagery is a journey in your mind to a relaxing place. Just concentrate on a mood and a place away from your present situation. Don't think about your muscles as in other relaxation techniques. Create images that are peaceful and calming to you. Picture yourself in any relaxing place, real or imaginary: a warm, sandy beach; on soft pillows in front of a fireplace; or floating on clouds. Bring into your image sights, sounds, textures, tastes, colors, and scents that are relaxing to you. To be most effective during labor, you and your partner should talk about your favorite images or journey, so that key words or phrases can help you return to a relaxed state (see *Relaxing Images*, page 106). You are totally in control. Be creative.

Touch Relaxation

Touch relaxation is one of the most important tools a labor partner will use during actual labor. With pressure, kneading, rhythmic stroking, or counterpressure, he can help mom release tense muscles. Practicing these techniques now will teach mom to release to touch during labor. It will teach the partner how to touch, stroke, massage, and press in the most effective ways. Some women enjoy and relax well to touch throughout labor. Others don't wish to be touched at all at certain times. Talk about your needs and use your own techniques during practice and actual labor.

Gentle Pressure — As contractions increase in intensity, you may notice tightening of the brow, eyes, jaw, or hands. Gentle pressure, with or without movement, can help her identify and release that tension. For overall tension – give her a strong bear hug and let her release into you.

Kneading — Slow rhythmic kneading is helpful for reducing tension in the shoulders, thighs, or buttocks. Grasp the muscle between the heel of your hand and your closed fingers. Squeeze in with gentle pressure, hold, then release and repeat, moving across the muscle. The thumbs may be used with the heel of the hand, but avoid pinching with thumb and fingers.

Stroking — Hand-over-hand stroking is effective on the back, thighs, or lower abdomen. Use firm pressure with the palm of the hand to stroke from shoulder to hip, or thigh to knee. Before one hand leaves the body, the other hand begins a second stroke. Alternate hands, maintaining constant contact with mom as you slowly move across her back or thigh. Hand-over-hand strokes across the lower abdomen may be done by mom during a contraction – it is a natural response to rub where it hurts.

Encircling the arm with two hands at her shoulder, squeeze gently, moving down the arm to the tips of the fingers with one long continuous stroke. Use the same technique from upper thigh to the toes. She will release her tension to your touch if her limbs are fully supported or her arms are hanging by her side. Do not drop her arm or leg as you release the fingers or toes.

Counterpressure — This sustained, generally heavy pressure is effective on painful areas of the lower back. Fold your fingers flat against the palm of your hand. Keeping the wrist straight, use the knuckles of that fist to press against her pain. Position yourself so your body will lean into your arm to increase the pressure from your fist. The heel of the hand may be used for counter pressure, but it's more uncomfortable on the wrist for long periods.

Sample Exercise

Frown ... *release* as partner strokes across forehead with fingers, or lays palm across it

Clench teeth ... *release* to pressure of palms cupping jaw or to stroking of jaw

Tighten arm ... *release* one muscle group at a time – biceps, forearm, hand, and fingers as partner strokes with two hands encircling arm

Clench fist ... *release* fingers as partner opens fingers and squeezes or massages hand

Hunch shoulders ... *release* to kneading or downward pressure of hands on shoulders in rhythm to each breath out

Arch back ... *release* to steady pressure or massage

Pull in abdominal muscles ... *release* to hand-over-hand stroking on lower abdomen

Tighten legs ... *release* to long stroking of the thighs, calves, and feet

Putting It All Together — *Total Body Release With Practice Contractions*

After you have learned all these relaxation techniques, you should be able to release your whole body on command. Progress from being able to relax in the ideal environment to letting go of tension while standing at the kitchen sink or sitting at a desk. Try as you may, you will not have a distraction-free environment during labor! When your partner says "contraction begins," make it a verbal cue to relax and breathe. Your partner should be alert for possible signs of tension and use the tools of verbal cues ("Relax your jaw"), visual imagery ("Remember the warmth of the beach"), and touch to encourage relaxation. A pain stimulus such as holding a hand in ice water can be used to simulate a contraction. As you continue to practice and master the various relaxation techniques, you will notice improvement in your ability to cope with "practice contractions."

Womb Mates

Giving birth to multiples – twins, triplets, or more – is certain to multiply the joy to parents. However, along with added joy comes added risk and added precaution. When two or more babies share a womb, it expands to make room for them–and so must mom. It is amazing what a body can do. But as you might expect, many of the challenges of pregnancy are multiplied along with the increase in size and number of babies.

Moving with care is important when the center of gravity is so changed by a large abdomen. With added weight, more stress is put on the back. Sturdy flat heeled shoes and a maternity girdle may help to ease discomforts. Pelvic tilts on hands and knees may move the babies and relieve an aching back.

The heart is pumping more blood to flow through additional placentas. More amniotic fluid is required for more than one baby. Because of this, circulation exercises are important to help prevent swelling of tissues and varicose veins. Plenty of fluids are necessary to stay well hydrated and help prevent preterm labor.

At 32 weeks the size of the uterus with twins is about the same as it is for a singleton at term of 40 weeks. There is not much to do to prevent stretch marks, but using a massage oil over the enlarged abdomen feels good and may help relieve itching.

Low birth weight, prematurity, and the positions in the womb are the most common problems for babies in multiple births. Anemia and preeclampsia are possible complications for the mother. Testing is performed frequently in the last trimester to avoid these problems. Ultrasounds are done to keep check on growth and amniotic fluid levels. Non-stress tests check heartbeats in reaction to movement. There are tests that can be done to check for possible preterm labor. Over half of twin births occur prior to the 37th week. For triplets, closer to 92 per cent are born by that time. Fortunately, multiples develop faster than singletons, and their lungs tend to mature sooner.

Bedrest is a common recommendation, especially for higher order multiples. While not all studies agree on the benefit of bed rest, it is obvious that mothers of multiples need lots of rest. Fatigue sets in earlier. Most complications occur by 30 weeks, so good weight gain and plenty of rest even in early pregnancy is important. The high cesarean birth rate is being challenged for twins as it is for single babies. Some believe that infant breathing problems may be increased without the stimulation of a vaginal birth. But many factors play a part in this decision.

Labor for multiples is usually shorter than labor for a single baby, but in some cases a uterus is so stretched that contractions are inefficient and labor is slow. Birth may be easier because the babies tend to be smaller than singletons. Twins' average birth weight (5 pounds, 5 ounces) is about 2 pounds less than the average single baby (7½ pounds).

To give your babies the very best start in life, eat a well-balanced diet with adequate calories and protein, and drink lots of water. Keep prenatal appointments to check blood and urine, weight gain, and blood pressure. Reduce your stress through time management and relaxation practice. To reduce fear and anxiety, prepare for birth, and talk to other parents of multiples. This advice is no different than for other pregnant couples - it's just doubly or triply important!

Multiple Facts

- The natural occurrence of twins is one in 89 births.
- Asian countries have the lowest twinning rate.
- Identical multiples occur when one fertilized egg splits into two or more identical sections which develop separately.
- Fraternal twins are formed from two eggs and two sperm (instead of one which splits) and can look just as similar or different as any siblings.
- Identicals have similar foot and hand prints, but different finger prints.
- About one quarter of identical twins are "mirror" twins. Features such as birthmarks and hair whorls appear on opposite sides of each twin.
- Having multiples in the family on the father's side does not increase the chance that his children will be multiples, but it could pass to his daughter for her to carry the tendency to the next generation.
- Heaviest twins: 14 pounds and 13 pounds, 12 oz. in 1924; 10 pounds, 14 oz., and 12 pounds, 3 oz. in 2008.
- Lightest living twins: 1 pound, 4 ounces and 8.6 ounces born in 2004 at 25 weeks, 6 days gestation.
- Earliest premature triplets with all to survive: 2 sets born at 24 weeks in 2002 and in 2005.

(For a copy of *Preparing for Multiples - The Family Way*, contact www.thefamilyway.com or 713-528-0277.)

Ideas for Preparing Siblings

- Read books about babies and talk about what new babies are like. Role play with dolls what changes might occur in the family. If the child seems interested, use books to answer questions about "where babies come from."

- Get out the older child's baby book and look at it with him. Show how you cared for him when he was a young baby (a lot of time rocking, holding, nursing, etc.).

- If possible, borrow a young baby for a day to let the older child see what it is like to interact with the baby.

- If you are planning a school, room, or bed change for the older child, do it as early in your pregnancy as possible so the older child doesn't feel "kicked out" by the baby.

- Encourage the older child to help you get things ready for the baby.

- If the child is mature enough, let him go with you to the doctor to listen to the baby's heartbeat. Look at books together that show the growth of the baby.

- Begin preparing the older child for the separation if mom will be in the hospital or birth center. Show him where mom will be. If he will be spending the night away from home, you might let him have a practice run.

- Enroll your child in a sibling preparation class.

- Record stories that can be played while you are in the hospital or birth center or busy with the baby.

- Pack a new T-shirt that says "I'm a big brother (or sister)." Whoever is keeping your older child can give it to him as soon as the new baby is born.

- Call your older child after the new baby arrives to tell him the good news (unless it's during the night). Don't be disappointed if he is not quite as excited as you are – it takes time!

- When you come home from the hospital, let daddy carry the baby so your arms are open for your older child.

- Let the older child hold and help with the care of the baby as much as possible.

- Ask visitors to greet the older child and pay attention to him before greeting the baby.

- Read a story to the older child while feeding the baby.

- Plan a special time each day for just you and the older child.

- Expect some "acting out" or regressive behavior from the older child. After all, his adjustment to the new baby is at least as great as your adjustment to your first baby. What is really needed is lots of love and the reassurance that the new baby is not taking his place.

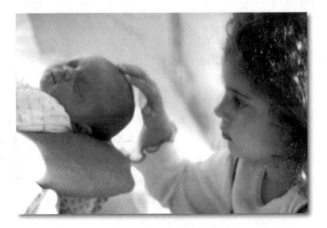

Recommended Reading to Prepare Siblings

Recommended for baby to preschool age:

Civardi, Anne, Michelle Bates, & Stephen Cartwright. *Usborne First Experiences the New Baby.*

Cole, Joanna & Maxie Chambliss. *When You Were Inside Mommy.*

Falwell, Cathryn. *We Have a New Baby.*

Kubler, Annie. *My New Baby* (New Baby Series) (pictures only, no words)

Falwell, Cathryn. *We Have a Baby.*

Repkin, Mark, Judy Torqus, and David Moneysmith. *Mommy Breastfeeds My Baby Brother.*

Scott, Ann Herbert & Glo Coalson. *On Mother's Lap.*

Metropolitan Museum of Art & Marie Madel Franc-Nohain. *My New Baby and Me: A First Year Record Book for Big Brothers and Big Sisters.*

Recommended for ages 4 to 8:

Bernhard, Emery & Durga Bernhard. *A Ride on Mother's Back: A Day of Baby Carrying around the World.*

Corey, Dorothy & Nancy Poydar. *Will There Be a Lap for Me?*

Frasier, Debra. *On the Day You Were Born.*

Gordon, Judith, Vivien Cohen, & Sol Gordon. *Did the Sun Shine Before You Were Born?* (facts of life)

Hoban, Russell & Lillian Hoban. *A Baby Sister for Frances.*

Keats, Ezra Jack. *Peter's Chair.*

Lansky, Vicki & Jane Prince. *A New Baby at Koko Bear's House.*

Mayle, Peter. *Where Did I Come From?*

Nilsson, Lennart & Lena Katarina Swanberg. *How Was I Born? A Child's Journey Through the Miracle of Birth.*

Rogers, Fred. *The New Baby.*

Sears, Martha, William Sears, Christie Watts Kelly, & Renee Andriani. *Baby on the Way* (Sears Children Library).

Sears, William, Martha Sears, Christie Watts Kelly, & Renee Andriani. *What Baby Needs* (Sears Children Library).

Recommended for parents:

Faber, Adele & Elaine Mazlish. *Siblings Without Rivalry: How to Help Your Children Live Together So You Can Live Too.*

To Be Or Not To Be . . . Concerned

When visiting a care provider (doctor, nurse, or midwife), mom is checked for such things as high blood pressure, anemia, diabetes, and preeclampsia. The baby is checked for heart tones, movement, and growth. Take a list of questions or concerns with you – it may save you a "panic call" later.

At times you may feel that the normal symptoms of pregnancy such as fatigue, urinary frequency, and back pain are just "different." You can trust your body to give you warning signals if problems arise. Take time to listen to those signals and to contact your health care provider if something seems wrong.

Throughout your pregnancy your uterus will contract from time to time. Learn to recognize this so you won't miss the signal if your body warns you of possible preterm labor. Early recognition of a preterm labor may prevent a premature birth, so do not ignore or deny the signals. Learn to feel your contracting uterus by pressing and releasing the muscle with your fingers. Sit comfortably relaxed or lie on your side and begin to feel your belly starting at the navel, moving down the center, across to the sides, and back up to the navel. The uterus is contracting if it feels firm to the touch, like touching your forehead.

Trust your instincts. If you feel that something is not quite right with you or your baby, that is the time to be checked. On the other hand, remember that many of the "signals" given below can occur normally in pregnancy as well. Some swelling, occasional dizziness, increased discharge or urination, ligament pain, backache, gas pains, "spotting" following sex or exam, pressure from baby's weight, and contractions are all a normal part of pregnancy. It is up to you to decide if what you feel is a change from your normal experience of pregnancy. If so, ask the advice of your nurse, doctor, or midwife.

To ease your concerns eat well, drink plenty of fluids, nap or relax each day, and spend time "talking" to your baby. After the fifth month of pregnancy, you may want to count your baby's movements periodically (see page 98).

Signals of preeclampsia	Signals of infection	Signals of problems with the placenta
• Persistent or severe headaches • Excessive dizziness • Blurred vision • Excessive swelling • Sudden, rapid weight gain • Protein in urine • Increased blood pressure	• Fever • Vaginal discharge with foul odor • Pain or burning with urination • Decreased amount of urine	• Sharp, persistent abdominal pain • Bleeding from vagina • Change in usual pattern of baby's movements and kicks (see page 98)

Signals of possible preterm labor	If signals of preterm labor occur	Call your Dr. or midwife immediately if
• 6 or more contractions per hour • Low, dull backache • Menstrual-like cramps • Intestinal cramps or diarrhea • Unusual pressure in pelvis, lower back, abdomen, or thighs • Water or large amounts of mucus leaking from the vagina • Red, pink, or brown vaginal discharge • Same signals as for labor, except they occur prior to 37 weeks of pregnancy	• Stop what you are doing • Empty your bladder • Drink 4 glasses of water (32 oz.) • Lie down on your left side for one hour • Feel contractions as described above *If you experience 6 or more contractions per hour before 37 weeks of pregnancy, call your health care provider. Often times the signals will weaken or disappear with rest and fluids.*	• Vaginal bleeding occurs • Bag of waters breaks • Uterus contracts 6 or more times per hour before 37 weeks of pregnancy • Major change in baby's movement • Any of your body's signals are of concern to you

Childbirth

Women are as nervous and unsure of themselves as ever, and they need to learn to trust their bodies. Birthing is much more than eliminating pain. It is one of life's peak experiences.

Elisabeth Bing

Labor Support—Then and Now

Web It!

Stories of birth have always passed from woman to woman. Some tell memories of feeling love and support, while others remember being alone or afraid.

Turn of the 20th Century

A century ago the word "pregnancy" was hardly spoken in public. It was said that a woman was in a "delicate condition," or she was "in the family way." Her baby's birth usually took place in her home. She was attended by a midwife, surrounded by women to support her. As the century moved on, birth began to be seen as a medical event, rather than a normal life event. Doctors began to replace the midwife, and more births moved to the hospital. It was then that other women and family members were left out, and the woman labored alone with the aid of "twilight sleep" (morphine to reduce the pain and scopolamine to remove the memory of pain).

Mid-century

The negative effects of these drugs and the resulting forceps deliveries caused concern. Dr. Grantly Dick-Read brought in the idea of teaching women about the birth process as a way of reducing fear and pain. His thoughts were echoed and added to by such people as Drs. Fernand Lamaze, Robert Bradley, and Frederick Leboyer, and women advocates such as Marjorie Karmel and Elisabeth Bing. These people established programs to include the husband as "labor coach," allowing him to be present during birth to support his wife. Some men eagerly take this role, but others are extremely reluctant!

The 21st Century

The pendulum continues to swing. Pregnancy is spoken of freely, and active pregnant women are seen everywhere. Birth is often seen on the big screen and on the Internet. The husband or partner is valued for loving support and encouragement more than for active instruction. In many regions, women have a choice of birth locations and of people to support them during the birth. A husband, partner, family member, friend, doula, nurse, midwife, and/or physician may have a special role in helping to bring a baby into the world.

The Labor Doula

A professional labor assistant, or doula, is now an important member of the childbirth team. Doctors, labor nurses, and midwives often must care for more than one laboring woman at a time. A doula supports only one woman throughout her labor. A doula does not replace the partner in any way. She helps him support the mother, and guides the couple as they labor together. While the father-to-be will most likely want to be present for the birth of his baby, he doesn't always feel comfortable being the only support for his partner. Most often, he has never been at a birth before and may not have the knowledge and confidence that everything is going just as it should, even when it is. A doula assists the labor nurse in making suggestions for comfort and in giving encouragement and reassurance to the mother or couple. It is her continuous presence, along with her touch, knowledge, and experience with birth that makes her a valuable addition to the birthing team.

Several studies have found that mothers accompanied to labor by a doula had fewer cesarean births, shorter labors, fewer requests for pain medication and anesthesia, less need for oxytocin to stimulate labor, and less need for forceps to assist birth.

The role of a doula is not new, but the studies showing her value are. We are living in the best of times when we can offer the high technology of this century for research, emergencies, or complications while holding on to the high touch skills of women helping women with birth as they did over a century ago.

> Research shows that women who were supported by doulas during labor reported:
>
> - labor and birth as less painful
> - feeling more in control of birth
> - less anxiety after birth
> - feelings of increased self confidence
> - a lower incidence of postpartum depression
> - increased incidence of breastfeeding at 6 weeks
> - improved relationships with their partners
>
> *The Doula Book* by Klaus, Kennell, and Klaus.

How Long Will Labor Last?

This is the question most often asked, but impossible to answer. During pregnancy, women often hear stories about labors that last anywhere from less than an hour to over 48 hours. Fortunately, both extremes are rare. Each labor and birth is unique. Even different births of the same mother may vary greatly.

Most women don't begin labor with the cervix closed. Pre-labor contractions soften and begin to open the cervix. Some dilate several centimeters before labor begins. For this reason, it isn't known exactly how long it takes the cervix to dilate from 0 to 10 centimeters. Many experts say that an "average labor" for a first baby is anywhere from 12 to 17 hours. It takes about half that time for following births. They don't say how far the cervix has opened when that labor begins, though. A study published in *Obstetrics and Gynecology* reported that it takes an average of 7 to 8 hours for the cervix to dilate from 4 to 10 centimeters in a normal labor (when there is no medical intervention). Second stage takes a little less than one hour.

Sometimes the move from home to birth location can cause the contractions to slow down or stop for a while. This is normal. It's also common for labor to stall at some point. If your cervix has dilated several centimeters before true labor begins, your labor may be short. If your water breaks, or true contractions begin when the cervix is closed, you may have a longer labor. The length of a normal labor has a wide range.

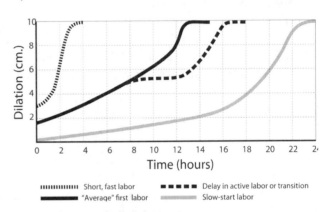

What will affect the progress of labor?

- ❧ How the baby fits in mom's pelvis
- ❧ The position of the baby
- ❧ The position and movement of mom
- ❧ Mom's confidence and the support she receives
- ❧ Medications and medical interventions used

Good news is that the longest phase of labor is also the easiest part. In this phase called "Early Labor" (see page 39), contractions may start out as far apart as 20 minutes and last only 30 to 45 seconds. Very little time in each hour is spent feeling contractions. Even though 5 is halfway to 10, it takes much longer to dilate from 1 to 5 centimeters than it does from 5 to 10 centimeters. Just take one contraction at a time!

How to Time Contractions

Duration—beginning to end of one contraction
Frequency—beginning of one contraction to the beginning of the next contraction

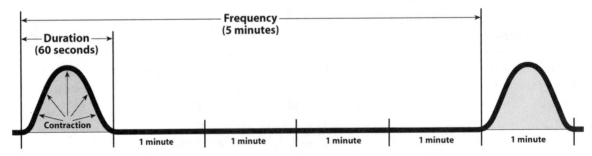

These contractions are coming every 5 minutes and lasting for 60 seconds

Normal Labor Variations

Short Fast Labor

A very short labor seems to be every woman's dream. However, short labors are not always easy labors. Contractions come on suddenly and are usually very intense. It is difficult to stay in control when your mind is expecting early labor contractions but your body is racing to 10 centimeters!

How to cope with a fast start of hard contractions:

- Get your mind where your body is – you may be closer to birth than your think.

- Breathe rhythmically.

- Keep eye contact with your partner.

- Follow Panic Routine if needed (see page 48).

- Move to side-lying position to help slow the birth.

Delay in Active Labor or Transition

Sometimes labor gets off to a normal start, but slows down after several hours. The size or position of the baby may cause a delay. If this happens, be active! Walking or swaying may help move the baby into a better position. If contractions are ineffective, augmentation (see page 49) may be needed.

How to cope if there is a long delay in progress:

- Walk!

- Change positions

    - Upright positions let gravity work

    - Sitting on the toilet may help the baby come down

    - Hands and knees or knee-chest positions may rotate the baby

- Shower or bathe to relax

- Use nipple stimulation if birth attendant agrees

- Listen to encouragement and support

- Have patience; give it time

Pre-labor or the Slow-start Labor

Some labors seem to take forever to get started. Contractions may come and go for hours or even days before the cervix finally begins to open. This is usually more discouraging and tiring than it is painful. Before a cervix can open, it must move forward, soften, and thin. This usually happens in the weeks before labor starts. But if it doesn't occur until mom feels the contractions, she will think she's "in labor" long before she really is. Have patience. Relax so that you are well-rested by the time active labor finally "kicks in." After the cervix dilates to 3-4 centimeters, labor usually moves in a timely fashion. But it can also begin slowly and continue as a long, slow-but-steady labor to the end.

How to cope with a slow-starting labor:

- Stay in touch with your partner and/or your doula for emotional support.

- Continue your regular activities as long as contractions are irregular or start and stop without getting noticeably stronger. Go to work, watch a movie, eat and drink as you need, and sleep as usual for you.

Delay in Second Stage

When the cervix has opened to 10 centimeters, some but not all women have a short time when they don't feel contractions. This is normal. Enjoy it as a "rest and be thankful" phase. Upright positions, especially squatting, may trigger the urge to push. If epidural analgesia has been used, a mother will "labor down," waiting for the baby to come down when the time is right. If needed, forceps or suction may help with the birth.

How Painful Will Labor Be?

Pain during childbirth varies from one woman to another and from one birth to another. What you expect and what you fear, as well as your cultural and religious beliefs, all affect the pain you feel in labor. Contractions are sometimes called "labor pains," "rushes," or "surges." Whatever you call them, these contractions bring about the birth of a baby. The uterus is the largest and strongest muscle in a woman's body. When it contracts, there is a strong sensation of both pressure and stretching as this powerful muscle pulls back on the cervix to open the way to the birth canal. As the baby moves down the birth canal, more pressure is put on the other organs, and more stretching occurs. The pain felt varies from excruciating to mild. In a few instances a woman will say her labor was not painful at all. The length of labor does not always determine the degree of pain. Some short labors are extremely intense and painful while some very long labors are manageable throughout, and vice versa.

There are important differences between labor pain and other kinds of pain that women may feel in their lifetimes. Labor P-A-I-N is

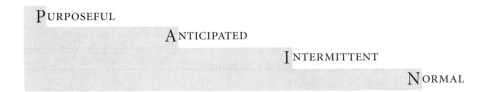

PURPOSEFUL

ANTICIPATED

INTERMITTENT

NORMAL

Labor Pain is Purposeful

It brings about the birth of a baby. Research studies show that laboring women who imagined holding their newborn babies in their arms reported less pain than those who concentrated on other thoughts. Sometimes pain in labor is giving a message to the laboring woman—empty your bladder, or change positions to relieve the pressure on your back. Labor pain also triggers the release of stress hormones in the baby, which prepare the baby for birth and for life outside the uterus. In the mother who has not had pain medication, the release of endorphins follows the intensity of the labor contractions. Endorphins are morphine-like substances made by the body to relieve pain. Long distance runners and athletes may also experience a purposeful pain and enjoy the "runner's high" caused by endorphins.

Labor Pain is Anticipated

Since you know to expect pain in labor, you can prepare yourself ahead of time by learning pain management skills. It is easier to manage pain that is expected than pain of unknown causes. For most women, labor contractions come in a regular pattern. During labor you will learn the rhythm of your contractions and be able to anticipate when the next one is coming.

Labor Pain is Intermittent

The rest period between contractions is one of the best-kept secrets of labor. Labor pain is not continuous like the pain of kidney stones or an abscessed tooth. Laboring women have a break between contractions to rest and regroup. During the final stages of dilation, the contractions may seem to come one on top of another, but an active partner, nurse, or doula can help you let go of the previous contraction and relax briefly before the next one comes.

Labor Pain is Normal

A woman's body was designed for pregnancy and childbirth. In most cases, labor and birth are normal processes, which do not involve illness or injury. Labor contractions are healthy, powerful sensations that push a baby into the outside world. In the same way that exercise enthusiasts, dancers, and athletes push their bodies to perform, many women choose to experience the full normal sensations of labor and birth, even though hard work is required. Some women describe unmedicated birth as a "peak" experience in their lives, increasing self-confidence for future challenges.

Labor pain is normal and natural, but today it is an option. Look at the Pain Medication Preference Scale on page 110 and decide where you fit on the scale. Then discuss your options with your health care provider.

You Will Be Better Able To Deal With Pain If You . . .

- Learn to think positively and overcome fear of birth. Good childbirth education with correct information helps to reduce fear of the unknown and fear caused by myths and stories. Listen to stories and read facts that will increase your confidence. Ask for information, and express your concerns to knowledgeable people during pregnancy and during labor.

- Find a support group for yourself. Surround yourself by people who care about you and who share a positive attitude toward birth with you. Decide what roles you wish for your family, friends, and birth attendants to play. Do not labor alone.

- Find a birth location where you may move freely. Ask if they have rocking chairs, birth balls, and extra pillows. If not, plan to take your own ball and pillows. Upright positions help with labor progress and comfort.

- Practice pain-management skills before birth. Massage, relaxation, and rhythmic breathing can all be used to reduce stress during pregnancy and to cope with contractions during labor. Learning these skills will give you confidence in your ability to labor. These same skills will help you deal with tension and stress throughout life.

- Try to enter labor well-nourished and well-rested. Everything hurts more when you are hungry and tired. Take care of your physical and emotional needs in the weeks before labor begins.

- Make your labor environment right for you. Adjust the lights. Play music. Relax in a warm tub or shower. Use scented bath oil and/or lotion. Aromatherapists say that lavender promotes relaxation, while jasmine has positive effects on labor progress and comfort. Experiment with scents before labor and use those you like. (See page 96 for suggestions of other things to take with you to labor.)

- Know your options for medications and medical procedures. What is available to you? What are the risks and benefits of your options? It is your choice whether you wish to work with the pain or ask your care provider to give you relief in the form of medication.

- Know that your partner will encourage you and suggest comfort measures other than medication unless you say your code word, e.g., "uncle." For those planning a natural birth, this prearranged code word will let your partner know if you no longer want to cope without medication. See page 110.

- Remember that pain in labor has a positive purpose. It is pain that you expect, just as an athlete does prior to a major event. Contractions come and go, so more time in labor is spent pain-free than in pain. Giving birth is a normal, natural event in the cycle of life.

For Better or For Worse®   **by Lynn Johnston**

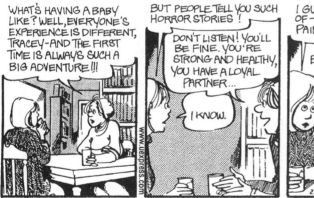
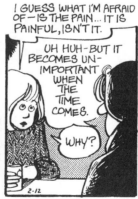
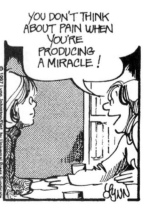

Signs of Labor

Sometimes labor begins before it is really expected, and sometimes it seems that labor will never begin. You may be "teased" by labor's beginning, then stopping, only to begin again on another day. Some women just experience labor in phases over days or even weeks. What is often called "false labor" is more accurately called "pre-labor." It may be causing the cervix to tilt forward, to soften, and to thin—three things that must happen to the cervix before it can open. If you think you are in labor, try the following: walk awhile, relax, shower or bathe, eat foods that are easy to digest, finish packing—then wait until your body tells you that things are "different" enough, or contractions are frequent enough (averaging 60 seconds in length, at five-minute intervals for an hour) to call your caregiver.

Signs of labor vary from one woman to the next and from one pregnancy to the next.

Sign	When It Occurs	What Happens	What Mom Notices	What To Do
Lightening *Engagement*	Two to four weeks before labor	Baby drops or settles into pelvis	Less pressure on stomach and lungs, more pressure on bladder	Wait for more signs of labor
Nesting	A day or two before labor	Impulse to clean or rearrange her "nest"	Sudden burst of energy	Be careful not to become overtired
Show	From hours up to a week before labor	Plug of mucus filling opening of cervix is released, as cervix begins to thin and open	Blood tinged mucous plug	Pack, stay well rested, and be ready when labor begins
Flu-like symptoms *(without fever)*	From hours to days before labor	Nature's way of cleaning out to make way for the baby	Diarrhea, nausea, or mild cramps	Rest, drink fluids, prepare for labor
Backache	Onset of labor and/or during labor	Contracting uterus pulls on lower back	Intermittent backache in time with uterine contractions	Relax, cold packs, heat (bath or shower), massage, positioning
"Bag of waters" leaks	May occur anytime from onset of labor to birth	Tear in amniotic sac causes fluid to leak out	Dampness or trickle of water to gush of fluid from vagina	Call caregiver to report: "*COAT*"–*C*olor, *O*dor, *A*mount, *T*ime; wear a pad or diaper to catch the leaks
Contractions	May occur anytime	Uterine muscles tighten	Weak to strong pressure or pain	Decide if true or prelabor; term or preterm

Pre-labor Contractions

- Generally tighten only portions of the uterus, rarely with back pressure
- Usually of short duration (15-45 seconds)
- Do not increase in intensity
- May not become closer together
- Usually irregular in occurrence
- Changing activity or position may make them stop
- Walking does not make them stronger

True Labor Contractions

- Generally tighten entire uterus and may be felt as back pressure or in low abdomen
- Duration becomes progressively longer (up to 60 sec.)
- Become progressively stronger in intensity
- Become closer together
- Most often become regular in occurrence
- Changing activity or position does not make them stop
- Walking may make them stronger

Stage One: Early Labor

What's Happening

Early labor contractions may start out as far apart as 20 minutes and last only 30 to 45 seconds. The cervix may have already moved forward, softened, and thinned to prepare for labor. If not, these changes will take place once labor begins.

For the easiest fit, the baby usually faces the mother's side as his head enters the top of the pelvis. During this phase the cervix will completely thin (efface 100%), and open (dilate) to about 4 centimeters. More of the mucous plug, or "show," may drop out as the cervix opens. Labor may begin with the bag of waters leaking. Usually, however, the membranes do not break until late in labor. Gradually the contractions become stronger and closer together. As labor moves to the active phase, contractions will be about 5 minutes apart and last up to 60 seconds.

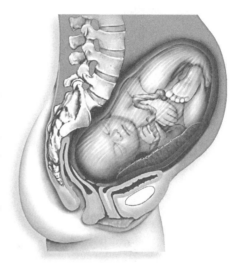

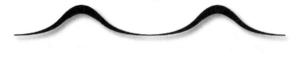

What the Laboring Woman May Feel	What the Laboring Woman Can Do	What the Partner Can Do
• Mild contractions (some women compare to menstrual cramps) • Backache • Mild diarrhea • Excitement • Anticipation • Relief that labor has begun • Happy • Some apprehension	• If labor begins during sleeping hours, try to rest for as long as possible. • Walk! • Change positions frequently, favoring upright positions. • Continue normal activities as long as possible, but do not over-exert – distract yourself. • Take a warm bath or shower – using a hand-held massager is helpful. • Rest! • Eat and drink lightly. • Try pelvic tilt for backache. • Begin focused breathing if needed. • RELAX!	• If labor begins during sleeping hours, encourage mom to rest for as long as possible. • Keep mom company – walk with her, play cards, watch TV, etc. • Encourage mom to change positions frequently, favoring upright positions. • Time *some* contractions and keep a written record. • Call health care provider as he/she has instructed. • Help mom relax! • Massage her back if it aches and suggest comfortable positions. • Tell her how well she is doing. • Put suitcases and pillows in car. • Make yourself a sandwich for goody bag and put in car.

Stage One: Active Labor

What's Happening

During active labor, the contractions continue to get longer, stronger, and closer together. They increase from 45 to 60 seconds long. They come every 5 to every 2 minutes apart. These stronger contractions open the cervix from about 4 to 7 centimeters. As the baby labors during this phase, he keeps his chin tucked. His body rotates to match the widest part of his head with the widest part of mom's pelvis.

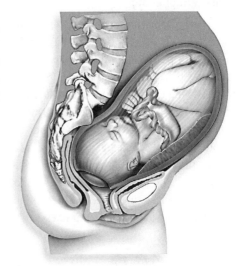

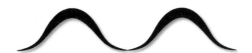

What the Laboring Woman May Feel	What the Laboring Woman Can Do	What the Partner Can Do

• Strong contractions
• Increased backache
• Growing seriousness
• Increasing concentration
• Desire for companionship
• Apprehension
• Uncertain if she can do it
	• Walk if comfortable.
	• Go to hospital/birth center.
	• Change positions often, favoring upright positions:
	  - lunge (page 47),
	  - lean or sway on a ball (page 21),
	  - rock in a rocking chair.
	• Try warm shower and/or bath.
	• Breathe slowly or in patterns.
	• Visualize holding the baby in your arms and/or visualize your "special place."
	• During pelvic exams, relax pelvic floor muscles.
		SUPPORT her:
		  Supportive environment
		  Urinate at least once an hour
		  Position changes frequently
		  Praise and encouragement
		  Out-of-bed (walk/shower)
		  Relaxation
		  Touch and massage
		• Eliminate distractions in the environment – add to comfort with pillows, dimmed lights, music, etc.
		• Keep lips and mouth moist.
		• Give back massage.
		• Do knee press or counterpressure (page 47).
		• Continue to tell her how well she is doing.
		• Change into scrub suit (if requested).

Stage One: Transition

What's Happening

Transition means change. In this phase of labor the powerful contractions that open the cervix change to the pushing contractions that bring the birth of the baby. Fortunately for most women, this is the shortest phase of labor. It only takes about 10 to 90 minutes for the cervix to open from 7 to 10 centimeters. Transition contractions may last 60 to 90 seconds. The time between them may be only 1 to 3 minutes. If the bag of waters has not broken earlier in labor, it will usually break during this phase. The baby completes turning to face his mother's back. He is then ready to begin the trip through the birth canal.

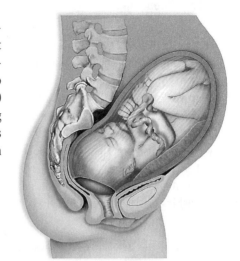

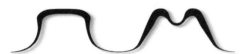

What the Laboring Woman May Feel	What the Laboring Woman Can Do	What the Partner Can Do
• Very intense contractions • Nausea and vomiting • Dozing between contractions • Mood change – irritable • Desire to give up, go home • Hot flashes • Chills and shaking legs • Heavy show • Severe low backache • Possible premature urge to push • Rectal pressure	• Experiment to find your most comfortable position. • Concentrate on the power of the contraction rather than the pain. • Visualize the cervix opening up and the baby moving down. • Take one contraction at a time. • Remember, this is the shortest phase of labor. • Use breathing patterns. • Relax and rest between contractions. • If an urge to push is felt, ask your nurse if small pushes might help labor progress.	• Encourage her to concentrate on the power of the contractions, rather than the pain, and to use visualization. • Remind her that this is the shortest phase of labor. • Remind her to take one contraction at a time. • Squeeze her hand or give her something to squeeze. • Breathe with her. • Apply counterpressure. • Give her a firm bearhug. • Put a cool washrag on her forehead if she is nauseous or hot. • Get extra blankets and massage her legs if she has chills. • Keep lips and mouth moist. • Help her to rest and relax between contractions. • Tell her how great she's doing and that baby will be here soon. • Tell her that you love her.

Stage Two: Pushing and Birth

What's Happening

The second stage of labor begins when the cervix is fully open (complete dilation). It continues until the baby is born. This may take from 15 minutes to 3 hours or more. Some women have a short resting phase between "transition" and "pushing" when the contractions are very mild. During this time the uterus is tightening around the baby's body after the head has passed through the cervix. When contractions return, they are farther apart than they were in transition. They come about every 3 to 5 minutes and last 60 to 90 seconds. Many women find the urge to bear down irresistible as the contraction builds. For most women, the sensations of pushing are less painful than the contractions of transition.

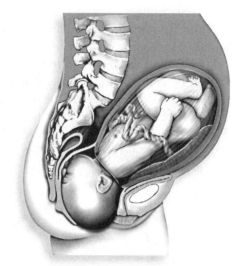

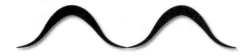

What the Laboring Woman May Feel	What the Laboring Woman Can Do	What the Partner Can Do

• Possible lull – up to 20 minutes while her body rests to get ready for the pushing stage
• Almost uncontrollable urge to push
• Very strong back and rectal pressure
• "Second wind" of strength to make pushing effort
• "Pins-and-needles" stretching sensations as baby crowns
• Exhaustion between contractions
• Relief that she can actively bring about the birth of her baby
• Ecstatic sensations as baby is born
	• Experiment to find your best position for pushing:
	  - semi-sitting
	  - side-lying (left)
	  - squatting (widens outlet)
	  - all fours
	• Relax shoulders, neck, legs, and jaw.
	• Use spontaneous or directed pushing as explained on page 44.
	• Relax perineum.
	• Open your eyes for the birth!
		• Help her to find her most comfortable and productive position.
		• Whisper words of encouragement: "You're doing just fine," "Just like that," "Just perfect."
		• Encourage her to rest between contractions.
		• Explain pushing preferences to your nurse so she can work with you.
		• If she prefers to hold her breath while pushing, remind her to breathe every 6-10 seconds.
		• Remind her to relax perineum.
		• Remind her to open her eyes to see the birth.

Stage Three: Delivery of the Placenta

The placenta separates from the uterus and is pushed out through the birth canal in 5 to 20 minutes.

What the Laboring Woman May Feel	What the Laboring Woman Can Do	What the Partner Can Do
• Mild contractions • Joy • Fatigue • Relief that baby is here	• Gently push as you feel the urge or as instructed by birth attendant. • Take slow, deep breaths.	• Greet the baby as he or she is placed on mom's chest.

Breathing Strategies for Labor

Some women go through labor and birth, breathing naturally, without using any special breathing strategies. Others focus on slow breathing to help them relax, or on special breathing patterns for a distraction during contractions.

Breathing Awareness

Become aware of your normal breath. Place one hand on your upper chest and the other on the lower curve of your belly. Feel the movement in your chest, belly, or both as you breathe in and out.

Another way to focus on your breath is for your partner to place both hands in various places on your back – the low back, middle, then upper back. Focus your attention on the warmth and pressure of the touch and breathe towards it.

Slow, focused breathing has been used in meditation and yoga practices for centuries. It has been shown to reduce stress, both in labor and in life. As you relax, your breathing naturally slows. By consciously slowing your breathing pace, you can help yourself release tension. Concentrating on a focal point in the room or closing your eyes to focus inward may help you become more in tune with your breathing.

Breathing Pace and Patterns

We normally breathe in and out without thinking. However, some women find that focusing on the depth and pace of each breath helps them to "ride" over the peak of the contraction. Bring in new energy and blow away tension by taking a "cleansing breath." This is just a deep breath – like a natural sigh you use each day. In labor you may choose to begin and end each contraction with a cleansing breath. Through the contraction you will breathe to the depth, pace, and pattern that feels right to you. Many women focus on a slow, relaxed pattern throughout labor. Others choose to change the breathing pace and/or pattern as the contractions change. While breathing at a slow pace is generally more relaxing, varying the pace or pattern is often a good focus or distraction. Most people are comfortable if they consciously pace their breathing at between half and twice their own normal breathing rate. Throughout labor you should breathe in the way most comfortable for you: in and out through the nose; in through the nose and out through the mouth; or in and out through the mouth.

Strategies to Accompany Breathing

Visualize scenes such as

- an ocean wave slowly rolling in as you inhale; slowly rolling out as you exhale.
- being surrounded by your favorite relaxing color, breathing in that color to spread its relaxing effects to all of your body; then breathing out a color of tension.
- the soft petals of a flower gradually opening up as the morning sun strikes.
- your cervix opening, opening, opening to the full 10 centimeters. (Use this only when you are in labor.)

Repeat rhythmical phrases such as

- "Breathe in for my baby, breathe out tension."
- "Breathe in energy, blow away pain."

Count

- *to a number:* count to 4 or 5 as you breathe in; and the same number or more as you breathe out.
- *your own pattern:* inhale and exhale a certain number of times, ending each pattern with a soft blow (3 to 1 pattern – breathe in, out; in, out; in, out; in, soft blow). See page 107. The labor partner can suggest changing patterns during the contraction by signaling with his fingers or voice a pattern for mom to try.

Whisper words or sounds on exhalation such as

- "hee" or "huh." (Keep mouth, lips, and jaw relaxed.)
- "hee" or "huh" a certain number of times, then give a soft blow or "huu" (example: "hee, hee, huu").

Combine

- *different paces:* breathe slowly at the beginning and end of the contraction, and faster over the peak.
- *imagery and counting:* visualize a group of lighted candles, counting them as you blow them out.
- any of the strategies above.

Strategies for Second Stage

It isn't always easy to tell just when second stage begins. Some women experience a lull after the cervix has dilated to ten centimeters. This rest period may let the baby move deeper into the pelvis while the laboring woman gathers strength for pushing. Other women feel an urge to bear down before the cervix is completely dilated. There are times when small, natural pushes may help labor progress, and other times when active pushing should wait.

If epidural analgesia has been given, a woman may not feel her body's urge to bear down, even when her cervix has completely dilated to 10 centimeters. Research studies show that it's best to rest without actively pushing, until the uterus alone pushes the baby down to +1 station, or the top of the baby's head can be seen. After this period of "laboring down," an urge to push is usually felt by the mother and either spontaneous or directed pushing can begin.

Spontaneous Pushing

Spontaneous pushing is used when the mother feels strong pushing urges. She responds by bearing down according to what she is feeling. Rather than counting or loudly calling out directions, her support team remains silent or whispers words of encouragement.

- Find the position most comfortable and efficient for you. A squatting position may increase the urge to push.
- Remember – you are using only your abdominal (voluntary) and uterine (involuntary) muscles for pushing, so position yourself so you can release the muscles in your arms, shoulders, legs, and face.
- Breathe as you like as the contraction builds. When you feel the urge to bear down, tune in to your body and push as you feel the need. Rest or take another deep breath as needed.
- You may make "birthing" or "grunting" sounds while slowly exhaling with the bearing-down effort.
- Push as often as your body tells you across the peak of each contraction.

Directed Pushing

Directed pushing is used if the mother is anesthetized, if the baby is coming down too slowly, or if hospital routine dictates. A mother with an epidural will probably not be directed to push until the baby has moved down to +1 station, or until the head can be seen.

Strategies to Consider

- If your caregiver tells you not to push, you may need to blow or "puff" repeatedly when you feel your body starting to push.
- If you feel you are not pushing effectively, ask your labor attendant to put a gloved hand or a warm compress on your perineum so you can feel the direction to push. A mirror placed so you can watch your progress when you push may also encourage and direct you.
- Try to imagine what is happening inside your body by visualizing your baby moving down the birth canal.
- When you feel a strong burning, stretching sensation, you will know your baby's birth is near. Try to release the pelvic floor muscles and concentrate on your baby.
- Partners can provide support by whispering encouraging phrases such as, "Just like that," "Good work," and "The baby's almost here."

Skin-to-Skin Contact Immediately After Birth

In most cases, you can expect that your baby will be given to you to hold skin-to-skin on your chest immediately after birth. This is a recommendation from the American Academy of Pediatrics and other experts. Holding your baby this way will help stabilize his breathing, heart rate, and temperature. Amazingly, the temperature of your chest will either increase or decrease to warm or cool your baby as needed. Checking your baby and giving an Apgar Score can be done while you are holding your baby. Most babies are awake and alert immediately after birth. Left together, your baby will gradually find your breast and begin to nurse. Giving your baby time to self-latch in a relaxed and unhurried environment, and being skin-to-skin with you, will be most helpful in getting breastfeeding off to a good start.

Positions for Second Stage

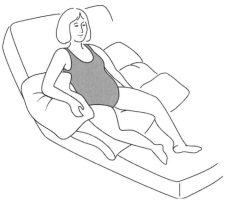

Pushing from the abdomen, with the upper body somewhat relaxed, will be less tiring.

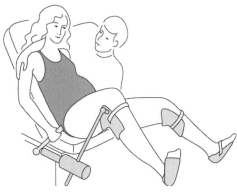

Semi-sitting is the most common position for birth, especially if an epidural is in place. Stirrups may or may not be used.

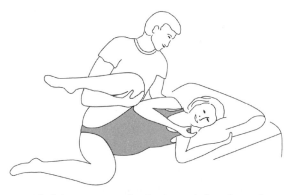

Side-lying may ease backache and slow down the birth in a short, fast labor. It may reduce pressure on the perineum to help avoid an episiotomy.

Being on hands and knees may help rotate a baby from the posterior to the anterior position and relieve pressure on mom's back.

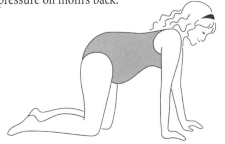

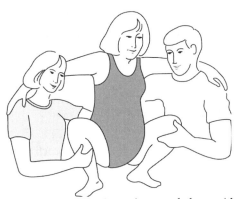

Squatting may help to widen the pelvic outlet and encourage a large baby to come down.

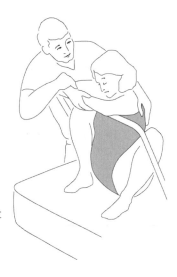

Possible Challenges of Labor

Challenge	Solution
Nausea	• Take slow, deep breaths. • Lie on left side or try sitting up. • Apply cool cloth to face. • Remember, nausea can be a sign of transition.
Chills/shakes	• Put on socks. • Add warm blankets and/or heat pack. • Use concentration and focal point. • Contract, then release all muscles. • Try other relaxation techniques such as visual imagery. • Do friction rub. • Partner give her a bearhug.
Leg cramps	• Partner place heel of affected leg in palm of his hand and use arm to gently push ball of foot toward mom's head. • Flex foot with toes towards head, or stand/walk on the leg. • Apply warm blankets or compresses.

Back pain
 	
Baby in posterior position puts pressure on spine
	• Change mother's position – get the baby off her spine (see pgs. 20-23):
	  – Side-lying with uterus tilted toward bed, pillow between knees
	  – Sitting up with back rounded
	  – Sitting up on side of bed with arms supported on bedside table
	  – All fours (on floor, over back of bed, over ball)
	• Try movement to encourage baby to rotate to an anterior position
	  – Pelvic tilt on all fours (page 16)
	  – Walking up and down stairs
	  – Standing or kneeling lunge (page 47)
	  – Abdominal lifting (page 47)
	  – Knee press (page 47)
	• Apply counterpressure (pages 16, 21, 23)
	  – Partner's hand
	  – Massage toy, small paint roller, or tennis balls in a sock
	• Apply heat or cold
	  – Warm shower or bath
	  – Ice packs or cold compresses
	  – Heating pad/hot water bottle, microwave heat pack

To make a reusable heat pack: Put 3 cups of uncooked rice in a cotton tube sock. Sew or tie the top closed. Microwave for 2 to 3 minutes for warm, moist heat.

Movements for Labor

Web It!

1. *Mom:* Stand facing forward with chair at your side. Place one foot on the chair, with toes and bent knee pointing straight to the side. Weight is on the straight leg.

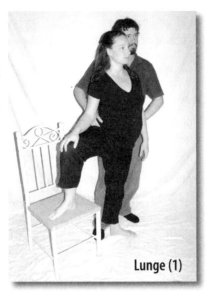
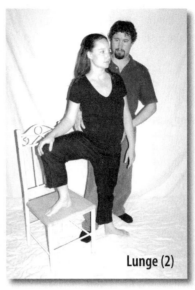

Lunge (1)

Lunge (2)

2. *Mom:* Lunge sideways, shifting weight to the chair, but don't let your knee go beyond your toes. This may open the pelvis to help baby rotate. Shift weight back to starting position. Repeat. Lunge in the direction that feels better.

Partner: Be near her to help her balance.

Abdominal Lifting

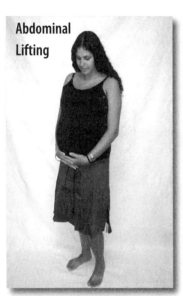

Mom: Stand with knees soft. Interlace your fingers and place under your belly. Lift your abdomen up and slightly in as you tilt your pelvis. This may relieve pressure and help lift the baby into a better position.

Note: Other pelvic tilt positions to relieve backache are pictured on pages 16 and 21.

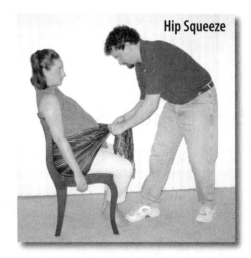

Hip Squeeze

Mom: Sit with rebozo (shawl) or sheet around your hips.

Partner: Pull on the rebozo, squeezing her hips together. This counter-pressure may relieve backache by releasing pressure on the ligaments in the pelvis during or between contractions.

Knee Press

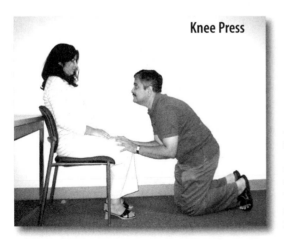

Mom: Sit in a chair that is braced against a table or wall so it won't slide. Sit up straight, with hips against the back of the chair.

Partner: Kneel, cupping your hands over her knee caps. Lock your elbows into your body while leaning forward into her knees. Your weight presses the long thigh bones into the hip joint to relieve pain in her back. Apply pressure gradually during each contraction, and release as the contraction ends.

What To Do If The Laboring Woman Panics

Many women ride every contraction of their labor with seeming ease and poise. However, many more feel that some contractions overwhelm them – that they "lose control" or "panic" and call out for help. The support person can help prevent this panic in some instances or help the mother regain control by being familiar with the "Panic Routine."

Pre-Panic Signals	Role of Partner
Restless or agitated body movements	When you see tension: • Stroke it away with both touch and verbal signals ("release where I touch you, release to my hands"). • Apply back pressure if needed. • Talk it away ("Uncurl your toes," "I'll hold your hand," "Take a cleansing breath"). • Use phrases from your "special place" to encourage relaxation.
Unrhythmical, loud, or irregular breathing	Breathe with her. Start with her pace and slow it if necessary.
Loss of focal point *Eyes darting about or head moving side to side*	Keep your face close to hers. "Look at me."
Verbally giving up *"I can't do this anymore!"*	She is asking for your help. Acknowledge her pain. Reassure her, praise her, take charge. Try to get her to focus on the power of the contraction rather than the pain. See if you can get her to visualize the cervix opening up and the baby moving down. Use as much of the "Panic Routine" (below) as needed.

Panic Routine for Labor Partner

1. *Establish eye-to-eye contact* – Put your face in front of hers so she can see you. You may need to stand up.

2. *Hold her firmly* – Take either her hands, shoulders, or face in your hands to focus her attention on you.

3. *Breathe with her* – Tell her to breathe with you. Breathe loudly or use words or soft blowing into her face so that she can easily follow you. Begin at her pace and guide her to slower, quieter breaths as she follows you.

4. *Reassure her* – After the contraction is over, remind her that she can do this and you will be there to help her. Remind her that each contraction brings her closer to the birth of her baby. Words of encouragement and support from you, the nurse, and your caregiver can give her confidence in herself.

Childbirth Choices

Some pregnant women feel comfortable with the idea of a high-tech birth, while others want as "natural" an experience as possible. Think about the birth you want ahead of time. Talk about your choices with your care provider. Policies and procedures vary from one hospital to another, and from one doctor or midwife to another. Understanding the benefits and risks of common procedures and medications will help you make informed decisions. While labor and birth don't always go as planned, knowing your choices and being flexible will help you to have a positive birth experience.

Induction

Induction is the process of starting labor by artificial means. It shouldn't be done as a convenience for the pregnant woman or the doctor. It should only be done for medical reasons such as: membranes leaking for too long without contractions, a pregnancy lasting longer than 42 weeks, a mother with high blood pressure or other medical problems, or a baby who is not growing well or showing signs of stress. According to experts, including the American College of Obstetricians and Gynecologists (ACOG), suspecting even a very large baby is not a medical reason for induction. Research studies have shown that inducing for a big baby increases (rather than decreases) the chance of cesarean birth. For first-time mothers, inducing labor for any reason approximately doubles the risk of needing a cesarean delivery.

Health care providers in Canada discourage elective induction altogether, while new guidelines from the Joint Commission (the organization that accredits hospitals in the U.S.) discourage elective induction or scheduled cesarean surgery before 39 weeks.

Labor may be induced by putting a prostaglandin gel or other medication on the cervix to make it ripen (soften and open). Artificially rupturing the membranes (*amniotomy*) or the intravenous (IV) use of oxytocin (Pitocin) are other ways to induce labor. Breaking the water or an oxytocin drip might be used to increase (*augment*) contractions in a stalled labor if changing position, walking, or nipple stimulation doesn't help. If oxytocin is used, labor is monitored continuously with an electronic fetal heart monitor to assure that the baby isn't under stress. Induced contractions are often stronger and/or more frequent than natural contractions, needing more coping techniques.

Non-Stress Test, Biophysical Profile, and Stress Test

Before inducing labor, some physicians do a *non-stress* or a *stress test*. During a non-stress test, an external fetal monitor is attached to the mother's abdomen. The doctor studies the baby's heartbeat when the baby is moving. If the heartbeat is fine, the mother is allowed to go home and wait (usually another week) for labor to begin on its own. If the heartbeat shows that the baby should be born as soon as possible, then labor is induced or a cesarean birth occurs. A biophysical profile combines the nonstress test and ultrasound. The baby's breathing movements, muscle tone, body movement, and the amount of amniotic fluid are checked during the *biophysical profile*. During a stress test, contractions are induced with oxytocin while the baby's heartbeat is watched on an external electronic fetal monitor. If the heartbeat looks strong and healthy, the mother is allowed to go home and wait (usually a week) for labor to begin on its own. If the test indicates that the baby should be born very soon, then the oxytocin is continued and/or increased for an induction, or a cesarean birth occurs.

Fluids by Mouth/Intravenous Infusion (IV)

In a long labor, women need fluids so they don't become dehydrated. In many hospitals and birth centers, laboring women are encouraged to take fluids such as ice chips, popsicles, water, and other clear liquids by mouth. Others require fluids to be given through an *IV*, which is a plastic tube inserted into a vein in the hand or arm. An IV may also be used to give medication or for emergency procedures. It may be uncomfortable or more difficult to move around with an IV in place, but with a rolling IV pole, it is possible to walk, taking it along. Some caregivers wait until late in labor, when most women stay in bed, before starting a required IV. Another choice is to substitute a heparin lock, which holds a vein open without the attachment to an IV bag and pole until fluids or medications are needed. If your labor is induced with oxytocin or if you choose to have epidural anesthesia, an IV will be necessary.

Monitoring Fetal Heart Tones

According to experts such as the World Health Organization, ACOG, and the Association of Women's Health, Obstetric, and Neonatal Nurses (AWHONN), there are several safe and effective ways to monitor the baby's heartbeat during labor.

Intermittent Auscultation: Caregivers use a specially designed stethoscope (fetoscope) or a hand-held electronic device (Doppler) to listen to the baby's heartbeat on a set schedule. Between checks, the laboring woman is free to be up moving, showering, or walking without being connected to a monitor.

Electronic fetal heart monitoring (EFM): This is a method of measuring and recording the baby's heartbeat along with the mother's contractions. A monitor is attached either externally by two belts around the mother's belly or internally through the vagina to the baby's scalp and to the uterus. The internal monitor is more accurate and comfortable than the belts, but the bag of water must be broken to use it. Monitor leads may be detached or belts removed if EFM is used intermittently or used only for a baseline reading. However, it is often used continuously throughout labor. Monitor cords limit movement, but a woman is not always confined to bed. She may sit in a rocking chair, use a birth ball, or stand and sway nearby the monitor. Telemetry, a way of monitoring without cords attached to the monitor, is available at some hospitals. If the belts are waterproof, the laboring woman can take a bath or shower while being monitored.

For most mothers, continuous monitoring is not required unless oxytocin or an epidural is used. In some high risk pregnancies, it may be beneficial to have a constant reading on the condition of the baby throughout labor. Because there is wide variation in the way that fetal heart rate patterns are interpreted and because continuous monitoring is associated with an increase in risk for cesarean birth, the American College of Obstetricians and Gynecologists (ACOG), states that either continuous electronic fetal monitoring or intermittent auscultation is acceptable in a patient without complications. In Canada, obstetricians routinely recommend intermittent auscultation rather than continuous electronic fetal monitoring.

Amniotomy

Breaking the bag of waters by using an amnihook is called an *amniotomy*. This is sometimes done to see the color of the amniotic fluid (meconium-stained fluid may indicate fetal distress) or to induce or augment labor. Contractions may get closer together and stronger after amniotomy, thereby possibly shortening some labors. Intact, the bag of waters cushions the baby's head and reduces the chance of bacteria reaching the baby and the uterus. Once the membranes are ruptured, either on their own or by amniotomy, many health care providers feel that the baby should be born within 24 hours to reduce the chance of infection.

Episiotomy

An *episiotomy* is a surgical incision of the perineum, made to enlarge the vaginal opening at birth. This makes more room for the birth of a large baby or for the use of forceps. A local anesthetic is given so that the episiotomy repair is not painful, but most women report some pain after the anesthetic wears off. The length of recovery time varies among women. Some caregivers believe that it may help to avoid an episiotomy if massage is used to help stretch the perineal tissues during pregnancy. Neither ACOG or SOGC recommend routine use of episiotomies.

Forceps/Vacuum Extractor

Forceps or a *vacuum extractor* (suction device) may be used to help during a difficult birth. Both tools are used to speed up the second stage if the baby needs to be delivered quickly or if the mother can't push effectively due to anesthesia, exhaustion, or the size of the baby. An episiotomy is required when forceps are used. Forceps may cause bruises on the baby, which generally fade in about 48 hours. The suction may cause a little swelling, but this too soon disappears.

Circumcision

Circumcision is the surgical removal of all or part of the foreskin of the penis. Sometimes it is done for cultural or religious reasons. In the hospital setting, it is not done automatically on all boys, but is an operative procedure which requires the informed, signed consent of the parents. The American Academy of Pediatrics (AAP) says that the benefits of circumcision are not significant enough for the AAP to recommend circumcision for all newborn baby boys. Instead, they recommend that parents discuss the benefits and risks of circumcision with their baby's health care provider, and then make an informed decision about what is best for their child. The AAP also states that if parents decide to circumcise their infant, it is essential that pain relief be provided.

Management of Labor Pain

Sensations of uterine contractions have been described by laboring women as anything from "pressure" to "intense pain." Some women don't realize they are having contractions until birth is about to occur, yet others report labor pain for days before birth. Just as women's perceptions of labor pain vary, so do women's choices about pain management. Your choices regarding comfort measures and pain medications may depend upon the intensity and length of your labor; your own fears, concerns, and plans; the options available at your birth location; and the support you receive during labor.

Your own natural resources and education may provide the relief you need. Changing your position often, walking, slow dancing, and doing the pelvic tilt may reduce pain, as well as help the baby to come down. Warm baths and showers, massage, relaxation, and breathing techniques, along with the body's endorphins (morphine-like pain inhibitors which our bodies produce in high levels during an unmedicated labor), allow many women to cope with labor pain and to experience positive sensations of birth.

Studies have shown that the presence of a doula for physical and emotional labor support has significantly shortened the length of labor and reduced the pain perceived.

Narcotics and tranquilizers reduce pain and tension, whereas regional anesthetics (spinal and epidural blocks) numb the sensations of contractions and birth (pages 52-53). These choices provide pain relief for women who don't want to cope with the pain of contractions. Discuss your options with your health care provider. Learn about their advantages and side effects so that you will be fully informed.

Epidural Analgesia

Epidural analgesia is the most popular form of pain relief used by laboring women in North America. It causes some loss of feeling (numbing) in the lower half of the body, which relieves pain during labor and vaginal or cesarean birth.

Before an epidural is started, fluid is given through an IV in the vein of the hand or arm. The woman is placed in a curved position on her side or sitting up. A small area of skin on the lower back is numbed with local anesthesia. A needle is then placed through this area into the epidural space, which is located near the spine. A small plastic tube (catheter) is placed through the needle and the needle is withdrawn. The catheter is taped to her back, with one end remaining in the epidural space and the other end attached to a syringe of medication. The catheter remains in place throughout labor and birth, so that small amounts of anesthetic can be injected intermittently, either manually or by an electric pump. During a cesarean birth, higher doses are given. The amount of numbing depends on the drug and dose used. Low doses are less likely to cause side effects in mother or baby, according to ACOG. The medicine injected will affect the nerve fibers to the lower body, giving complete to partial pain relief. With a traditional epidural, the motor fibers are numbed, making movement of the legs difficult and walking impossible. Sometimes narcotics are injected alone or in combination with the numbing medications. These narcotic epidurals or "walking epidurals" give less numbing, allowing greater movement and possible walking. The pain relief experienced is usually not as great as with the traditional epidural. Narcotic epidurals are not available in all hospitals.

Epidural analgesia provides the most effective pain relief available for labor and birth, but it can have side effects. The mother's blood pressure may drop, which can cause the baby's heart rate to slow. This can usually be avoided by administering approximately a pint of IV fluid before the epidural is given.

ACOG states that labor may be prolonged 40 to 90 minutes with epidural analgesia, and there is approximately a twofold increased need for oxytocin augmentation. Increases in the length of the second stage of labor and a possibility of not feeling the urge to push contribute to higher use of forceps and vacuums in women with epidural analgesia. There is also an increased incidence of fever during labor.

If the laboring woman develops a fever, the baby may be tested after birth to make sure that the mother's fever was caused by the epidural, rather than by infection. These tests can lead to separation of mother and baby and delayed initiation of breastfeeding. With epidurals there are fewer effects on early behavior and readiness to breastfeed than with systemic narcotics.

Other complications are rare. If the covering of the spinal cord is punctured when the needle is placed, the mother may develop a severe headache which may last a few days. If the dose of numbing medication used for epidural analgesia unintentionally enters the spinal fluid or a vein around the epidural space, other serious complications may develop, such as difficulty breathing or rarely seizures. All of these events are rare in experienced hands.

References:
1. ACOG. 2002. *ACOG Practice Bulletin #36: Obstetric Analgesia & Anesthesia.*
2. ACOG. 2004. *ACOG Patient Education: Pain Relief During Labor and Delivery.* (Developed in conjunction with the American Society of Anesthesiologists)

Medications Available During Labor and Birth

STAGE I LABOR – Systemic drugs (affect the whole body)

Type of Drug	How Given/When Given	Duration	Purpose	Possible Effects on Mom	Possible Effects on Baby	Possible Effects on Labor
Barbiturates *(sleeping pills)* Seconal Nembutal Amytal	By mouth, IM (into muscle), or IV (into vein). IM medication crosses placenta within 5 minutes; IV within 1 minute. Generally given only in very early labor.	Seconal: 4-6 hrs Nembutal: 4-6 hrs Amytal: 7-8 hrs	• Often given to distinguish true labor contractions from pre-labor contractions • To promote rest and relaxation • Have no effect on pain	• Drowsiness • More difficult to focus during contractions • Nausea • Large doses: hypotension (low blood pressure), decreased pulse rate, and disorientation	• Respiratory depression • Decreased responsiveness • Decreased sucking ability • Hypotonia (decreased muscle tone) *Most pronounced if given within 4 hours of birth*	None known
Analgesics/Narcotics Demerol Nubain Stadol Sublimaze	Demerol: IM or IV Nubain: sub-Q (injected just under skin), IM, or IV Stadol: IM or IV Sublimaze: IM or IV *Note: Some analgesics/narcotics are now being given through the epidural catheter.* Generally given only in active labor.	Demerol: 2-3 hrs Nubain: 3-6 hrs Stadol: 3-4 hrs Sublimaze: 1-2 hrs	• To "take the edge off" the pain • To raise the pain threshold • To reduce pain (central nervous system depressant)	• Drowsiness • Disorientation • More difficult to focus during contractions • Hypotension • Nausea/vomiting • Dry mouth • Dizziness • IV: respiratory depression	• Respiratory depression • "Sleepy" baby • Decreased sucking ability *Most pronounced if given within 1 to 3 hours of birth*	• Can slow down labor • Need for additional medical procedures (continuous monitoring of fetal heart rate, IV)
Tranquilizers Valium Phenergan Vistaril Largon	IM or IV	Valium IM: 2-3 hrs Valium IV: 1-1½ hrs Phenergan: 6-8 hrs Vistaril: 4-6 hrs Largon: 3 hrs	• To reduce tension and anxiety • To relieve nausea • To relax muscles • To enhance effects of narcotics	• Drowsiness • Difficulty concentrating • Dry mouth • Hypotension	• "Sleepy" baby • Decreased responsiveness • Slow adaptation to feeding	None known
Inhalation Anesthesia Nitrous oxide *Note: Entonox combines 50% nitrous oxide and 50% oxygen in a cylinder. Nitrous oxide is used in many countries, but only at a few hospitals in the U.S.*	Self-administered (under supervision of dr./midwife): The laboring woman is given a facemask or mouthpiece attached to a gas mixture of nitrous oxide & oxygen. When she needs pain relief, she takes in a deep breath. The gas is "on" only when she is inhaling from the mask. May be used in both first & second stage.	Takes effect approximately 50 seconds after she begins taking the deep breath. Effects are very short-term.	To "take the edge off" the pain *Note: Pain relief provided is limited compared to epidural analgesia, but probably better than that provided by narcotics.* *About 50% of laboring women report satisfactory relief; 20% some relief; and about 30% report no pain relief at all.*	• Dizziness • Disorientation/confusion • Nausea • Claustrophobia if someone else tries to "help" by holding the mask on the laboring woman's face (not recommended)	None The gas does pass easily through the placenta to the baby, but it is rapidly eliminated as soon as the baby cries and starts to breathe. It does not have any effect on the fetal heart rate or circulation, or the baby's breathing at birth.	None

STAGE I LABOR – Regional Anesthetics (only affect one portion of the body)

Type of Drug	How Given/When Given	Duration	Purpose	Possible Effects on Mom	Possible Effects on Baby	Possible Effects on Labor
Epidural • "caine" drug • narcotic (such as Fentanyl) • "caine" drug + narcotic	Given in active labor while sidelying or sitting. Needle introduced into epidural space (not spinal fluid) and catheter left in place for continuous administration, or in case additional medication is needed.	Takes about 30 minutes to administer. Duration depends on drug used and method of administration (continuous or intermittent).	To relieve painful sensations of contractions, birth, and episiotomy repair To allow mom to be awake and alert Can be used for forceps/ cesareans	• Low blood pressure. • Incomplete coverage • 3% failure rate for epidural • Fever • Itching if narcotics used • Need for urinary catheter • Increase in perineal lacerations if forceps used	• Low blood pressure in mom can cause drop in fetal heart rate • Septic workup if mom has fever • Some medications used may impact early breastfeeding, requiring additional patience and assistance	• IV fluids and continuous electronic fetal heart rate monitoring required • Increased length of labor • Increased need for oxytocin augmentation • Higher incidence of operative vaginal deliveries (vacuum, forceps)
Intrathecal Narcotics (within spinal canal) Sufentanil Fentanyl Demerol Morphine	During active labor, a narcotic is injected into the subarachnoid space (space containing the spinal fluid) Utilizes a smaller needle than used for epidural analgesia	• 90-120 minutes • May be repeated, but offers much shorter period of pain relief	For rapid onset of pain relief No effect on motor function May not provide adequate pain relief for second stage (see combined spinal-epidural)	• May retain mobility • Able to feel urge to push • May cause itching, nausea, vomiting, urinary retention, hypotension, and spinal headaches (1-2%), respiratory depression	• Some studies have shown fetal heart rate abnormalities, especially bradycardia (slow heart rate), while other studies have not • See epidural (above) regarding breastfeeding	• IV fluids and continuous electronic fetal heart rate monitoring required • Morphine may prolong labor

Combined spinal-epidural analgesia is given in active labor and is intended to continue through birth. When the intrathecal narcotic is given, an epidural catheter is placed to administer anesthetics after the intrathecal dose wears off. Although this procedure combines the effects of both intrathecal narcotics and epidural analgesia, the laboring woman will not be mobile and may not feel the urge to push.

STAGE II LABOR: Birth of the baby – Regional anesthetics (in addition to epidural, intrathecal narcotics, or combined spinal-epidural analgesia)
(Systemic drugs are not recommended because of possible adverse effects on baby when given near the time of birth.)

Type of Drug	How Given/When Given	Duration	Purpose	Possible Effects on Mom	Possible Effects on Baby	Possible Effects on Labor
Local – one of the "caine" drugs	Injection into perineum immediately prior to episiotomy, or after birth for repair	Takes effect in 5 minutes and lasts 20 minutes	To numb perineum for episiotomy and repair	None	None	None
Pudendal Block - one of the "caine" drugs	Injection into pudendal nerves via vagina immediately prior to birth, or after birth for repair	Takes effect in 2-3 minutes and lasts 1 hour	• To numb vagina and perineum • Used for forceps delivery	Eliminates "stretching" sensations	None, except with preexisting fetal distress	• Partial loss of urge to push • Relaxes perineum
Spinal/Saddle. Spinal provides anesthesia from breasts down. *Saddle* effects those parts which rest on a saddle.	Injection into spinal fluid given sidelying or sitting bent over with back bowed	Takes effect in 3-5 minutes and lasts 1½ - 2 hours	• To offer complete anesthesia for contractions, birth, repair • To let mom be awake and alert • Can be used for forceps and cesarean deliveries	• Hypotension • Spinal headache • Loss of bladder tone (need for catheter)	• Hypotension in mom can cause drop in fetal heart rate • More research needed regarding possible subtle behavioral alterations	• Contractions may be stopped • Urge to push is lost • Forceps needed

Emergency Birth

The most important thing to remember about emergency births is that they are almost always very fast, easy, and uncomplicated. The attendant needs to do little more than "catch the baby."

1. If there seems to be no time to make it to the hospital or birth center, call 911 or an ambulance so that trained personnel are on their way. If you are in the car when you know birth is about to occur, pull to the side of the road and contact emergency personnel to meet you there. Trained paramedics may also be available at the nearest fire station.

2. Try to help the mother relax as much as possible.

3. Encourage the mother to assume her most comfortable position for birth. This is often an upright position such as sitting, standing, or squatting. Side lying is another good choice for a fast birth.

4. Clean newspapers can be placed underneath the mother to act as absorbent padding. A clean sheet should be placed over the newspapers. A plastic sheet or shower curtain can be used under the padding.

5. If time and place permit, the attendant should wash his or her hands up to the elbows for about four minutes, or use an alcohol-based hand sanitizer.

6. As the baby's head is crowning, many mothers have a tendency to hold back on their pushing efforts for fear of tearing their perineum. You should encourage this. She should be instructed to blow repeatedly while the head is being delivered so that she does not add to the pushing efforts of the uterus. In addition, the mother or attendant should place one hand on the baby's head and apply very gentle counter-pressure to the head as it is coming out, so that the baby is born in a very slow, controlled manner. This will help prevent harm to the baby and to the mother's perineum.

7. As soon as the head is born, the attendant should check to see if the amniotic sac is still intact around the baby. If it is, there will be a thin, film-like covering over the baby. Break this with any clean, sharp item and gently wipe the baby's face. If a sharp item is not available, find an area where the sac is not against the baby's head (like around the ear or under the chin), and twist the bag to break it. If the cord is around the baby's neck, slip it over the head. Do not pull on the baby in order to deliver the rest of the body.

8. The baby's head will turn to one side, on its own. The shoulders will probably be delivered during the next contraction or two. The attendant should support the baby's head and encourage the mother to push to help with the delivery of the shoulders. Once the shoulders are out, the rest of the baby will slip out very quickly.

9. Once the baby is born, hold the baby with his or her head lower than the chest, so that any fluids or mucus swallowed during birth will drain out. Gently wipe off the baby's face. Avoid putting your fingers in his/her mouth, as that will make the baby swallow. If the cord is long enough, place baby on the mother's belly or chest.

10. Do not cut the cord. Wait until trained personnel arrive or until you can get mother and baby to the hospital.

11. If the cord is long enough to allow, put the baby to the mother's breast. The skin-to-skin contact will help keep the baby warm, and the baby's suckling will help the placenta to detach from the wall of the uterus.

12. Do not pull on the cord to help deliver the placenta. The placenta will come out, or its delivery can wait until you get to the hospital or birth center. If the placenta is delivered at home, put it in a bag to take to the hospital so the doctor can examine it.

13. If the baby is not already at the mother's breast, be sure to put the baby immediately to breast as soon as the placenta is delivered. The baby's suckling will stimulate the uterus to contract and help to prevent possible dangerous bleeding (normal blood loss following childbirth is less than two cups).

14. Use blankets over mother and baby to keep them warm and to help mother's "shakes."

CONGRATULATIONS!

Are All Cesareans Necessary?

Over the past 30 years the cesarean birth rates in both the US and Canada have risen dramatically. Many people believe that far more "C-sections" are being done than are necessary. Yet cesarean rates may continue to rise. Fewer women are having vaginal births after a previous cesarean. Some women are choosing cesarean birth for their first baby because they fear labor. Others fear problems in later life blamed on vaginal birth. A few studies have shown more short-term urinary problems after vaginal births than after a cesarean for some women. However the cause of the problems may be due to medical procedures such as vacuum or forceps delivery and episiotomy, rather than normal vaginal birth. Until recently, episiotomy has been a routine part of most births, especially for first-time mothers. In 2000, the American College of Obstetricians and Gynecologists stated that, "ACOG does not recommend routine use of episiotomies." Fewer episiotomies may reduce those problems. Cesarean birth is major surgery. This means more risk of infection, blood loss, urinary tract or bowel injury, and blood clots. Recovery time is longer. It may be harder to get breastfeeding off to a good start. Because cesarean surgery increases risks in future pregnancies, elective (without medical reason) cesarean birth is not recommended for women who plan to have several children. According to the Joint Commission (the organization that accredits hospitals in the U.S.), delivery shouldn't be scheduled before the 39th week of pregnancy. Give yourself the best possible chance to avoid an unnecessary cesarean by doing these things during your pregnancy:

- Take good care of yourself with good nutrition and regular exercise.
- Arrange to have a doula or friend be with you and your partner in labor to provide continuous support.
- Discuss with your midwife or doctor what signs help them determine if a cesarean birth is necessary.
- If your baby is breech, and with your caregiver's permission, try the exercise below to rotate the baby.
- If your baby remains breech, talk to your caregiver about a procedure called external version.
- Read policies your doctor or midwife and your place of birth have for vaginal birth after cesarean (see page 59).
- Understand the use, benefits, and risks of medical interventions (see pages 49-53).

Give your labor the best chance of progressing.

- Let labor begin on its own. Avoid induction of labor unless there is a medical reason.
- Avoid epidural anesthesia in early labor.
- Walk through as much of labor as you can.
- Change positions frequently; avoid lying flat. If available, use a rocking chair or birth ball.
- Empty your bladder at least every hour.
- Relax in a warm bath or shower, if available.
- Listen to encouragement from your partner and medical team. Give your body time.
- Push with your body's urge in second stage. Try squatting if you have no natural urge-to-push or if the baby remains "high." If you have had epidural analgesia and don't feel an urge to push, ask for extra time for the baby to move down before you actively push (known as "laboring-down"). You can also request that the epidural medication be turned down or off during second stage.

Rotating a Breech

Dr. DeSa Sousa found this exercise to be 89% effective in her practice for rotating breech babies to a head-down position. Lie on your back with your knees bent and your hips raised 9 to 12 inches. Do this twice a day, 10 minutes each time, with an empty stomach and bladder. Use firm pillows under your hips to lift your pelvis. There is no known risk to mother or baby, so the exercise is worth a try if your baby is in a breech position after the seventh month of pregnancy. No studies have been done to prove that this exercise causes a baby to turn, but some report that it works.

Cesarean Birth

There are times when, regardless of what is tried, a cesarean birth becomes necessary. The safety of mother and baby is the most important consideration. The birth of a child, regardless of the path, can and should be a joyful, family-centered experience. If a cesarean becomes necessary, you will be more comfortable and confident if you know what to expect. During pregnancy, it is wise for all parents to discuss options with the doctor who would perform the surgery.

Generally, there are signs late in pregnancy or during labor that indicate the need for a non-emergency cesarean. The doctor and parents have time to discuss their options. Some of these signs include: breech or shoulder presentation; *placenta previa* (placenta completely or partly covering the cervix); active genital herpes infection; failed induction; baby's head won't fit through mother's pelvis (*CPD*); or an active labor which doesn't progress after many hours.

In rare cases an emergency cesarean must be done. Such problems as fetal distress, a *prolapsed cord* (cord comes down before the baby), or *placenta abruptio* (the placenta separates from the wall of the uterus before birth) could occur. A true emergency may call for emergency drugs and a quick mask with general anesthesia so the baby can be born within minutes. In this case the father or labor partner is usually not allowed to be present at the birth. Fortunately, emergencies are rare. There is time for regional anesthesia for most unplanned cesareans.

Options for a Non-emergency Cesarean

If you know ahead of time that you will have a cesarean birth, consider the following options that some women choose. Talk to your doctor about any that appeal to you.

- Wait until labor begins on its own, rather than scheduling the cesarean. A period of labor benefits the baby.
- Request to have your support people present at the birth.
- Be awake for the birth with epidural or spinal anesthesia. Learn about anesthesia options and how they are given.
- Discuss the sedatives given before surgery, which might make you groggy during birth.
- Ask for a transverse incision on the uterus. (The incisions on the skin and on the uterus may be different.)
- Request that your hands be free during the surgery to touch the baby as soon as possible after the birth.
- Request the screen be lowered just at the moment of birth so you can see the baby immediately.
- Decide with the anesthesiologist whether or not you need a sedative or pain reliever immediately after the birth. These might make you groggy or drowsy in the recovery room.
- If the baby has to go to the nursery for medical reasons, have father or labor partner go with the baby.
- Request that the baby be placed skin-to-skin on your chest immediately after the delivery. The baby can be dried and the initial assessment can be done while the baby is on your chest.
- Keep the baby with you as you are moved to the recovery room. Allow the baby time to gradually find the breast and self-latch. This initial bonding and breastfeeding time will occur while anesthesia is still in effect.
- Delay the infant's eye medication until after bonding time.

Procedures for a Cesarean Birth

Once the mother is admitted to the hospital, a number of things happen before the surgery begins. A urine specimen is collected and blood is drawn. Sometimes an enema is required. Clipping of some pubic hair may be necessary if the hair will interfere with the operation. An IV is started, a blood pressure cuff is put on, and a heart monitor may be attached. A preoperative sedative may be offered as an option. Most commonly a regional block, epidural or spinal, is given so the mother can be awake for the birth. After the anesthesia is given, a Foley catheter is inserted into the bladder. Usually the partner remains with the mother during most of these procedures until she is taken to the surgical suite. Depending on the hospital, he may be able to go in with her immediately, or may be instructed to wait until the staff is ready for him to come in for the birth. An anesthesia screen is placed in front of mom to create a sterile field and also to block the view of the surgery. The mother's abdomen is scrubbed and drapes are placed around the surgical site. She is checked for total coverage of anesthesia before the surgery begins.

The Surgery and Birth

The baby is usually born within five to ten minutes after surgery has begun. Sometimes, however, it seems like a long time as they set up before the surgery begins. If you are in this situation, consider your environment. You may want to have music playing, a pleasant scent from lotion or oil on your shoulder or wrist that you can sniff, your partner's touch on your hands or shoulders, a calm voice to remind you to breathe and relax, and a friendly face to focus on. Plan for this ahead of time.

During surgery it is not uncommon to feel tugging sensations in the abdomen, pressure in the chest, or light shoulder pain. You will hear the sounds of suctioning and will smell a "burning" odor as blood vessels are cauterized to stop bleeding. Don't hesitate to ask for reassurance from those around you if you have any concerns. Slow deep breaths may also help to relieve anxiety. After the baby is born, some doctors lift the uterus outside the abdomen to examine it, then replace it. Others do not think it is necessary to do this. You may experience nausea during the process if it is done.

If it is an option for you, ask that your baby be placed skin-to-skin on your chest right after birth. It takes about 45 to 60 minutes to repair the incision. This is an ideal time for the new family to be together to connect and to help this time pass more quickly. If mom cannot hold the baby until in the recovery room, then dad may take his turn in the delivery suite and hold baby near mom's head.

Recovery

The usual stay in the recovery room is one to two hours. In some cases the epidural catheter will be left in place for 12 to 24 hours to give pain medication. If not, ask for additional medication just before the catheter is removed. This will give you a comfortable hour or so in recovery with the baby. Most hospitals allow both labor partner and baby to stay in the recovery room with the mother if she is alert and wishes it. When the baby is allowed to remain in skin-to-skin contact on the mother's chest, usually the baby will gradually find his way to the mother's breast and begin nursing. Allowing the baby to self-latch in a relaxed and unrushed environment and keeping mother and baby together as much as possible are the best ways to get breastfeeding off to a good start. The nurse will frequently check pulse, respiration, and blood pressure. You will have vaginal bleeding (*lochia*) just the same as if your baby were born vaginally. The nurse will check the lochia and surgical dressing and may massage the uterus to make sure it is firm. Chills and/or fever occur commonly after regional anesthesia. A warm blanket sometimes helps with the chills. The IV and Foley catheter are usually left in for about 24 hours.

A cesarean birth is major surgery. Even if you are breastfeeding, you can and should take pain medication if you are uncomfortable. Remind your doctors you are nursing so that they can prescribe the right drug. Oral pain medications work better if taken for the first week on a schedule, such as every three to six hours or as ordered. This keeps a steady amount in your blood stream to control pain. Pressing a pillow against your abdomen will protect the area and make it hurt less as you move, roll over, cough, sneeze, or position the baby for nursing. It is important to move and walk as soon as possible to speed your recovery. Even with medications, you will be uncomfortable as you begin walking and caring for yourself, so move slowly. Plan to limit yourself to your personal care and caring for your baby for about six weeks. Keep visitors to a minimum so that you can rest.

After Surgery

Gas pains are caused by air that enters the body cavity during the surgery. Oddly, it is sometimes felt as soreness in mom's shoulders. Tell the nurse if this happens to you. Your doctor can order a medication to help move the gas out more comfortably. Walking as soon as possible also helps. Avoid carbonated drinks, large amounts of cold fluids, or using straws. Instead drink warm apple or grape juice to speed gas passage. A lighter-type diet is recommended at first. Avoid "heavy," fried, or gas-forming foods. Gently massage your abdomen in the direction of the natural clockwise flow of the large intestines to stimulate the gas to move. But avoid the area of the incision!

To speed your recovery, eat healthy foods, drink plenty of fluids, and rest often. Your physician may suggest these or other guidelines:

- No driving for several weeks, or at least as long as you are on pain medication.
- No housework or lifting for six weeks. Don't lift anything heavier than your baby (not a baby in a car seat).
- Sexual activity may be resumed when both internal and external incisions heal, vaginal blood flow stops, and you feel ready. This usually takes about six weeks. Personal lubricants are helpful at first.

Warning Signs after Surgery

Once home, report any of the following symptoms to your health care provider for further evaluation.

- Chills or fever
- Drainage from incision site
- Uterine tenderness
- Foul smell around incision
- Lower abdominal pains
- Increase in vaginal blood flow, color turning back to brighter red, passage of blood clots, or soaking a pad an hour needs to be reported immediately

Possible Emotional Feelings of Cesarean Parents

Some couples share only positive feelings of a cesarean birth, but many have some negative feelings. Talking about it with one another and knowing that other couples have felt the same way is helpful. You may also find it helpful to talk with someone from a cesarean support group.

Other parents have felt:

- Excitement at the birth of their baby
- Relief that it's finally over and baby is okay
- Anger at not being able to have a vaginal birth
- Anger if the mother had to have general anesthesia and/or the father or labor partner could not be present at the birth
- Estrangement from the baby if the mother was asleep or the father was not present at the birth
- Disappointment if the birth experience did not meet expectations
- Resentment at baby, father or labor partner, physician, or hospital staff
- Guilt that mother did something to cause the cesarean
- Worry about recovery period and scar
- Fear about future pregnancies and the need for future cesareans

Recovery at Home

Don't try to be superwoman! You are recovering from major surgery as well as the birth of a baby. Take it easy for at least two weeks, and plan to nap daily for at least six weeks. Your first priorities should be getting breastfeeding off to a good start and forming new family bonds. Get help with the housework so you can rest and spend your time with the baby.

- Keep supplies such as diapers, pitcher of water, and nutritious snacks close by.
- Use paper plates and cups for meals.
- Check with your physician regarding recommendations for bathing. Most suggest no tub baths until the steri-strips have been removed.
- Your incision may itch for many months. Warm compresses and gentle scratching will help.
- Limit visitors unless they come to help.
- Drink plenty of liquids and eat a well balanced diet.

Vaginal Birth After Cesarean – *VBAC – pronounced "vee-back"*

Web It!

If you have had a cesarean delivery, you and your health care provider will have to decide whether you will have a trial of labor (TOL) for a vaginal birth or a repeat cesarean delivery in your next pregnancy. At one time it was thought that once a woman had a cesarean, she should always have cesarean deliveries. However current evidence and experts such as the American College of Obstetricians (ACOG) and the Society of Obstetricians and Gynecologists of Canada (SOGC) recommend a trial of labor for a vaginal birth for most women who have had one previous cesarean delivery with a low transverse (horizonal) incision. You and your health care provider will have to balance the risks associated with vaginal delivery versus the risks associated with repeat cesarean delivery in your particular case.

Major surgery of any type brings with it possible complications such as blood clots and infection. If you have a repeat cesarean delivery, you are again at risk of these complications, as well as having risks of excess bleeding associated with complications of the placenta. In rare situations, the bleeding is severe enough to lead to the need for blood transfusions and/or the removal of the uterus (hysterectomy). Each cesarean increases risks of complications in future pregnancies, even if the surgery follows a trial of labor. If you choose to have a trial of labor (TOL) for a vaginal birth, a serious risk is uterine rupture. Statistics indicate, however, that the likelihood of this happening is about the same as that of a major complication occurring for a first-time mother.

In a practice bulletin issued in August 2010, ACOG broadened the number of women who may be candidates for TOL to include women with two previous low transverse cesarean deliveries, women expecting twins, and women with an unknown uterine scar type. ACOG also stated that the use of epidural analgesia and labor induction are options for women undergoing TOL.

VBAC is safest for women who go into labor on their own. For these women, the risks of a serious problem are about the same as for a woman with her first labor. A large study by the National Institutes of Health stated, "Overall the risk for a serious newborn complication is approximately 1 in 2000 trials of labor." This risk is due to the chance of the uterus separating or rupturing during labor. If the scar on the uterus separates, it doesn't normally cause problems. But if the uterus ruptures, it is dangerous for both the mother and the baby. A cesarean must be done immediately. If the uterus ruptures, the mother may have heavy bleeding and doctors may need to remove the uterus (hysterectomy).

With a vaginal birth, a mother has less risk of infection, blood loss, urinary tract or bowel injury, and blood clots. Recovery from vaginal birth is easier and faster than from surgery, so a mother is able to care for her newborn sooner. A baby who is born by vaginal birth that begins on its own has less risk of breathing complications and preterm birth. Breastfeeding success rates are higher for women who give birth vaginally than for those who give birth by cesarean. Costs of a cesarean birth are greater than those of a vaginal birth.

In 2010, a National Institutes of Health expert panel concluded that TOL is a reasonable option for many pregnant women with a prior low transverse (horizontal) uterine incision. The panel called for physicians and hospitals to make it possible for more women to have a trial of labor. Women who would like a vaginal birth after cesarean should discuss this with their doctor or midwife early in their pregnancy, to be sure that it will be an option for them.

*American College of Obstetricians and Gynecologists (ACOG). 2010. *ACOG Practice Bulletin 115 – Vaginal Birth After Previous Cesarean Delivery.*

Unexpected Outcomes

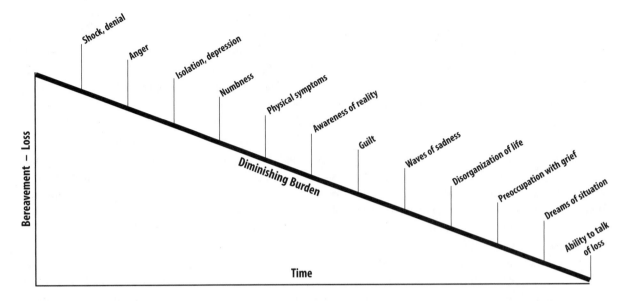

The Loss of a Dream

Regardless of the hopes and dreams we have about pregnancy and birth, there are no guarantees. For most, birth is a time of joy and relief, but sometimes when the unexpected occurs, it turns to a time of grief. Miscarriage or death of a newborn are obvious times of grief, but the cause for grief is not always death. Grief can be caused by a birth defect or injury, or even a birth experience that did not meet one's expectations. For some, a cesarean birth is a cause for grieving, if that possibility had not been included in the birth plan. The needs of a couple and the psychological adjustments that must be made are the same, regardless of the cause for grief, however insignificant the problem may seem to others. The "burdens" as outlined above may be passed through in any order. Time may be a matter of weeks, or may take many months or years. The time frame is rarely the same for all family members. Be patient with one another and realize that both anger and guilt are especially heavy burdens that can cause friction in a relationship. One may feel angry with the partner, who already feels guilty. This only magnifies the problem. Seek out others who have survived the problem that confronts you. Your nurse, health care provider, or childbirth educator may be able to put you in contact with an appropriate support group.

It is good to have a basic understanding of the grieving process, as grief comes to us all at some point in our lives.

- Understand the normal stages of grief.
- Grieve in your own way and time.
- Cry to relieve pain and tension. It is healthy.
- Express your feelings to your partner, and listen as your partner shares with you.
- Accept the fact that men and women may grieve in different ways.
- Locate a support group with others who have faced a problem such as you face.

The Loss of a Baby

If a baby dies, most parents are better able to cope with the loss if they have a chance to hold the baby and have pictures taken. Mementos such as a lock of hair, footprints, or an ID bracelet are helpful for parents to have for future memories. Naming the baby and holding a funeral or memorial service helps to bring the short life to closure. Final acceptance of a loss is hastened by an open discussion of feelings within the family or within a support group. Frequently there is another psychological upheaval on the anniversary date of the death.

Breastfeeding

Breastfeeding is not simply the transfer of milk from your breasts to your baby. It is also the transfer of smell, touch, warmth, and feelings as you and your baby gaze at each other...

Sue Cox

What Experts Are Saying About Breastfeeding

All over the world, health organizations promote breastfeeding to give babies the best possible start in life. According to the World Health Organization:

> "Breastfeeding is an unequalled way of providing ideal food for the healthy growth and development of infants.... As a global public health recommendation, infants should be exclusively breastfed for the first six months of life to achieve optimal growth, development, and health."

After six months, infants should receive appropriate foods while breastfeeding continues for up to two years of age or beyond.

Both the American Academy of Pediatrics (AAP) and the Canadian Paediatric Society (CPS) recommend exclusive breastfeeding for the first six months. The AAP recommends that breastfeeding continue for at least 12 months, and thereafter for as long as mutually desired; while the CPS recommends that breastfeeding may continue for up to two years and beyond.

In addition to the benefits of breastfeeding outlined in the following chart, studies have shown improved cognitive (brain) development and increased IQ scores in children and adults who were breastfed. The effect is greater with exclusive breastfeeding and longer breastfeeding durations.

Strong evidence exists that human milk reduces the incidence/severity of	A number of studies show a possible protective effect of human milk against	A number of studies indicate the following health benefits to the mother	Significant social and economic benefits to the nation include
Diarrhea	Sudden Infant Death Syndrome (SIDS)	Less postpartum bleeding and more rapid return of the uterus to pre-pregnant size	Lower incidence of illness in the breastfed infant allows parents more time for siblings and family, and reduces their absences from work and lost income
Respiratory tract infection	Diabetes		
Ear infections (otitis media)	Cancer in the lymphatic system (lymphoma)	Earlier return to pre-pregnant weight	
Bacteria in the blood (bacteremia)	Leukemia	Increased childspacing due to delayed resumption of ovulation (and menstruation)	At least $1000 to $2300 savings in formula costs per baby during the first year
Bacterial meningitis	Hodgkin disease		
	Overweight and obesity		
Urinary tract infection	High cholesterol	Less blood loss over the months following birth, due to lack of "periods"	Significant savings in health care costs due to fewer and shorter hospitalizations, fewer office visits, and decreased need for medications
Severe inflammation of the intestines and colon (necrotizing enterocolitis)	Asthma	Decreased risk of breast cancer	
In addition, postneonatal (after the first 4 weeks) infant mortality rates in the United States are reduced by 21% in breastfed infants.		Decreased risk of ovarian cancer	Decreased environmental burden for disposal of formula cans, bottles
		Possibly decreased risk of hip fractures and osteoporosis in the postmenopausal period	

Adapted from AAP Policy Statement, as reported in *Pediatrics*, Volume 115, February 2005

In addition to the many health benefits, nursing can become an easy and natural bonding experience for mother and baby. However, sometimes the road to this wonderful experience is a little rocky. Here are some hints based on recommendations from the American Academy of Pediatrics to help smooth the way:

- Healthy babies should be placed skin-to-skin with their mothers immediately after birth and stay there until the first feeding is finished.

- Except for unusual circumstances, the newborn should remain with the mother throughout the recovery period.

- Breastfeeding is made easier by rooming-in both day and night.

- Newborns should be nursed when they show early signs of hunger. These are rooting, hand-to-mouth movements, sucking on hand, small sounds, and small body movements. Crying is a late sign of hunger.

- The mother may offer both breasts at each feeding, but it is important that the baby finishes nursing on one breast before offering the second breast. Breastmilk changes during a feeding. A baby needs the higher-fat "hind-milk," which comes towards the end of a feeding. Some babies are satisfied by feeding from only one breast. If that happens, offer the other breast first at the next feeding, so that each receives equal stimulation and draining.

- No supplements (sugar water, formula, etc.) should be given to breastfeeding newborns unless ordered by a doctor for a medical reason.

- Mother and baby should sleep near to each other to make breastfeeding easier.

At the same time you are learning to breastfeed, you will have other challenges. The mother's physical discomforts following birth, fatigue of both mother and father, and learning to care for a baby 24 hours a day are challenging. Sometimes it seems easy to blame the baby's frequent crying and need for nighttime feedings on the lack of quality or quantity of mother's milk. In reality, most newborns, whether bottlefed or breastfed, have fussy periods and wake up during the night to eat! If you can answer "yes" to the checklist on page 69, you may be reassured that breastfeeding is going well.

Support and Encouragement

Mothers who receive support and encouragement to continue nursing past these first hectic weeks usually find that breastfeeding is very rewarding. While you are still pregnant, make a list of people you will call if you have questions or problems with nursing. This could be a sister or friend who has successfully breastfed her own child and will encourage you. Keep phone numbers for La Leche League, a lactation consultant, and your childbirth or breastfeeding educator. Learn as much as possible about breastfeeding. This will help build your confidence.

Frequent Feedings in Early Weeks

The more often you nurse your baby, the more milk you will make. Each time you put your baby to breast, your body sends out a hormone that causes you to make more milk. The way you hold your baby and the way the baby latches on to your breast make a difference in how effectively your baby nurses. If you put a baby on a strict schedule in the first months instead of nursing when he wants, you may not make enough milk. Newborns should nurse at least 8 to 12 times in 24-hours. This means the feedings will be from 1½ to 3 hours apart. Just like most adults, babies don't get hungry on a strict schedule.

Every few weeks babies go through a growth spurt when they seem to want to nurse all the time. To meet this increased need, nurse your baby more often when this happens. This will increase your milk supply. If you give supplemental formula during this time or at any time during the first few weeks, it can interfere with the supply-and-demand balance. If he gets formula, he won't be ready to nurse as often, so you will make less milk. Try to get some extra rest during growth spurts. They last only a few days before the feedings spread out again.

Avoid Bottle Nipples and Pacifiers

The sucking action of the baby's mouth on the breast is different from the way a baby sucks on a bottle. Many orthodontists agree that the sucking of breastfeeding helps to develop the jaw more completely. If given even a few bottles in the early days of life, some babies may develop "nipple preference" or "nipple confusion." They may refuse to take the breast, because it is easier to get milk to flow from a bottle nipple. Tell the nurses if you intend to breastfeed exclusively so they will not give the baby a bottle. The American Academy of Pediatrics and many lactation consultants discourage the early use of pacifiers for the full-term newborn. They want babies to meet their sucking needs at the breast until nursing is well-established.

Breastfeeding Guide

	What's Happening	What to Expect	What You Can Do
Prenatally	The pregnancy hormones in your body are preparing your body for breastfeeding.	• Your breasts gradually become larger, firmer, and more tender. • The brown part around your nipple (areola) becomes larger, darker, and develops small bumps called Montgomery glands. These glands are thought to secrete an antiseptic oil that decreases dryness. • Colostrum, a thick yellowish liquid, may or may not leak from the breasts.	• The good news is that there is very little that you need to do to prepare for breastfeeding; your body has already done most of the preparation and your breasts are completely ready to make milk by the 16th week of pregnancy. • Take a breastfeeding class. • Avoid using soap on the nipples, which may wash away the natural oils.
Immediately After Birth	The delivery of the placenta causes a drop in estrogen and progesterone, which stimulates initial milk production.	According to the AAP, the alert, healthy infant is capable of latching on to the breast without help within the first hour after birth. Being placed skin-to-skin on mother's chest and nuzzling at the breast are beneficial, even it it takes your baby longer than an hour to self-latch. You don't have to watch the clock. Research indicates that allowing your baby to find the breast and self-attach helps him learn to breastfeed sooner.	• Have the baby placed skin-to-skin on your chest and remain there until he or she has nursed. • Ask that the baby remain with you throughout your recovery period. • If you have a cesarean birth, ask that your baby be placed skin-to-skin on your chest during the surgical repair and the time spent in the recovery room. • Room-in, both during the day and at night. • Request night feedings if not rooming-in.
First Few Days After Birth	Your milk will come in.	• Your breasts may feel very full and heavy. • They may become engorged—firm and uncomfortable. This early engorgement will disappear spontaneously. • Nipples feel the most tender at this time.	• Watch your baby for early feeding cues and nurse often; newborns should be nursing 8 to 12 times every 24 hours. Wake the sleepy baby every 4 hours if necessary to get in the 8 to 12 feedings. • Offer both breasts at each feeding. • Learn different nursing positions. • If you are still in the hospital, continue rooming-in. • Once you are at home, try to get plenty of rest.
Ten Days After Birth	If you had engorgement, it usually has gone. Normal swelling of your lymph glands has also decreased, so that your breasts may actually feel smaller.	• Babies tend to be very fussy at about 10 days, about the same time engorgement stops; you may feel that you are not making enough milk. This is usually not the case; just a coincidence. • Nipple soreness should be gone by 10-14 days.	• Lie down to nurse, to get more rest. • Nap during the day when the baby sleeps. You still need extra rest! • Continue frequent nursings. Most newborns need at least 8 to 12 feedings every 24 hours. • Contact a lactation consultant if nipples are still sore at 10 to 14 days.
One Month After Birth	You are often resuming many activities you pursued before the pregnancy.	• Your baby may experience a growth spurt, needing to nurse even more frequently for 24-48 hours in order to build up your milk supply. At this age babies still tend to be fussy for many reasons other than hunger.	• You still need extra rest during the day. • Share your feelings (both positive and negative) with your partner and your friends. Do something special for you and your partner or just for yourself. • As long as your baby is gaining weight, be assured that he is getting plenty to eat! (Also, see page 69.)
Six Weeks After Birth	Hooray! Usually you are "feeling yourself" again and have recovered physically from the birth.	Your baby, too, seems much happier. He is starting to coo and smile often. He seems to have some kind of feeding pattern (although the pattern may change often).	• Keep up the good work! • Try to rest when you're tired. • Continue frequent nursings and *expect* some periodic growth spurts when your baby needs to nurse "all the time" in order to build up your supply of breastmilk. • Enjoy this very special time in your family's life.

Breastfeeding Challenges and Solutions

Challenge	Solution
Inverted nipples	• Babies nurse on the breast rather than just on the nipple. With a good latch, inverted nipples are not a problem for many babies. They are able to evert the nipple and nurse well. • If the baby is having difficulty latching on, you can bring the nipple out with a breast pump just before nursing. • If you continue to have problems, contact a lactation consultant.
Sore nipples	• Check your nursing position. Baby should be tummy-to-tummy with mother. Both the baby's chin and cheeks should be touching the mother's breast. Support the breast during feeding (see page 69). • Make sure more of the lower portion of the areola is in the baby's mouth than the upper portion. • Be sure to break suction before removing the baby from the breast. • Alternate nursing positions: sitting, lying down, or "football hold." • Nipples shouldn't hurt when you nurse. Pain is almost always caused by poor latch or positioning. Contact a lactation consultant and have her watch you nurse. • Begin nursing on the least sore side first. • Massage breast to stimulate let-down reflex before putting baby to breast. • Use relaxation techniques and slow breathing when baby first begins sucking and for as long as necessary. • End feeding when baby is finished; do not let the baby sleep at the breast when nipples are sore. • Air dry nipples after nursing. • Apply one of the following to the nipple and areola: warm, moist compresses; expressed breastmilk; hydrogel pads; or pure hospital-grade lanolin. • If using a breast pump, use the lowest setting that is effective. • Never use "bicycle-horn" type pumps or plastic bra liners.
Engorgement	• Room-in and nurse frequently (every 1½-3 hours). • Wear a supportive bra for comfort. • Take a warm shower or apply warm compresses, and hand-express milk to soften areola before nursing. • Apply cold compresses between feedings.
Plugged ducts	• Apply warm compresses, or soak in warm tub before nursing. • Begin feeding on affected side. • Get baby's chin as close as possible to affected area. • Do breast massage while nursing. • Try to eliminate causes such as too-tight bra.

Breastfeeding Challenges and Solutions

Challenge	Solution
Breast infection *Mastitis*	• Remove milk by continuing to nurse frequently, by hand expressing, or by using a breast pump. • Nurse with baby's chin as close as possible to affected site. • Go to bed and rest. • Take antibiotics prescribed by your health care provider. • Apply warm compresses to affected breast.
Baby "sleeping too much"	• Newborns *do* need to nurse at least 8 to 12 times in 24 hours. If your baby is not nursing this often, you will need to wake her every 4 hours to nurse. Try the following to help wake up your baby: unwrap and undress her, change her diaper, talk to her, gently move her up and down and sideways, put her hand to her mouth, express a small amount of breastmilk so that she can smell it. It is usually not necessary to wake a baby at night to nurse unless she is not gaining enough weight.
"Not enough milk"	• Most mothers make plenty of milk for their babies, even for twins or more. Use the checklist on page 69 to see if breastfeeding is going well for you and your baby. • Call a nurse where your baby was born, a lactation consultant, or your baby's health care provider. Weighing your baby is the best way to tell whether he is getting enough milk.
"Colicky" baby *Long periods of unexplained crying. Colic begins after the baby is two weeks old and usually ends by 16 weeks.*	• Respond to early feeding cues before baby cries. • Continue to breastfeed often; changing to formula often makes symptoms worse. • The warmth and comfort of holding baby skin-to-skin while rocking, nursing, or sleeping may calm both of you. • A warm bath or warm compress to the stomach may help. • Although the problem is usually not caused by mother's diet, if the fussiness continues, *avoid* eating one of the following, for one week at a time, to see if it helps: dairy products; eggs; nuts; wheat.

I'd like to breastfeed but I really want to lose weight quickly!

You may, in fact, lose weight faster as a breastfeeding mother than as a bottlefeeding mother, since making milk uses energy (calories). Strict dieting is not recommended for any new mother, whether breastfeeding or formula feeding, because of the physical and emotional recovery time necessary following birth. Breastfeeding mothers who combine healthy food choices with regular exercise usually experience a slow, gradual weight loss that is likely to be permanent.

Expressing Breastmilk

Many women who breastfeed today express and store breastmilk. This can be done by hand expression or with a breast pump. Expert advice from a lactation consultant can be very helpful, because it is important that the pump "fit" the mother properly. She can help you find what you need from many different types of pumps on the market.

An easy and inexpensive way to collect breast milk is by hand expression. To hand express, wash your hands with soap and water. Use both hands to massage your breast in a circular motion toward the nipple. Place your thumb and index finger on the *areola* (dark skin surrounding the nipple) about 1 to 1½ inches back from the nipple and press inward toward the chest wall, gently rolling the thumb and finger forward. Repeat until the milk stops coming; then change to another place around the areola.

Many nursing mothers use hand expression or one of the cylinder hand pumps for occasional pumping. Bicycle-horn type hand pumps shouldn't be used. They often collect bacteria and they are likely to stress the nipples.

Also for occasional use, you can use a battery-operated hand pump. Many of these pumps require the mother to turn the vacuum off and on, to create a suck-release cycle. Some models have settings that will adjust the strength of the vacuum but many don't. These pumps can irritate the nipples if they aren't used correctly. If you choose a battery-operated or electric hand pump, get one with automatic cycling.

For mothers who pump on a regular basis, a hospital-grade, automatic electric pump is recommended. These have an automatic suction and you can control the vacuum. They can be used with a double kit so that both breasts can be pumped at the same time. "Double-pumping" saves time and increases the amount of milk made. For information on renting or buying these pumps, contact your childbirth educator or lactation consultant.

Before expressing milk by any method, wash your hands, then use both hands to massage the breast in a circular motion toward the nipple. This will stimulate the letdown reflex and encourage milk flow.

Storing and Freezing Breastmilk

- *Refrigeration.* According to the American Academy of Pediatrics, you can store expressed breastmilk for a healthy newborn in a refrigerator for up to 48 hours. Other researchers believe that expressed milk is safe in a refrigerator for about five days. Different guidelines may apply for the preterm or ill baby; check with your baby's doctor for her recommendations. Put the milk in the refrigerator soon after collecting.

- *Containers.* The best kind of container for storage is a glass or hard plastic bottle. These will preserve the infection-fighting properties of the milk. Opaque containers protect the milk from sunlight, which may alter components in the breastmilk. The greatest loss of infection-fighting properties of breastmilk is with disposable plastic bags. This may not be a concern if the baby is taking most of her feedings from the breast. Glass or hard plastic bottles should be washed with hot, soapy water and air dried after each use, or washed and dried in a dishwasher.

- *Freezing.* If you have a separate home freezer unit that freezes to 0 degrees Fahrenheit (-18 Celsius), breastmilk can be frozen for 3 to 6 months. If you use a standard combination refrigerator-freezer with a separate door for the freezer, breastmilk can be frozen for up to 3 months. If you're collecting milk for a healthy newborn, you can collect a little milk each day and add it to the bottle or bag so it's frozen in layers. Before adding new milk to already frozen milk, chill the new milk in the refrigerator for several hours. That way it won't thaw the milk that has already frozen. For the preterm or ill baby, store or freeze each collection of milk separately.

- *Thawing.* To thaw the frozen milk, hold the bottle or bag under cold running water, then under lukewarm running water. Thawed breastmilk should be used within 24 hours. Always throw away any remaining thawed breastmilk that the baby does not take. Do not refreeze.

> **Place the milk in the back of the refrigerator where it is colder, rather than in the door.**
>
> **Always label the milk with the dates collected, and use the oldest milk first.**
>
> **Never use a microwave or stove to thaw or heat breastmilk.**

You Know Breastfeeding Is Going Well When . . .

_____ **You recognize your baby's early feeding cues:** Rooting, hand to mouth movements, sucking on hand, small sounds, and small body movements. Crying is a late feeding cue.

_____ **You can nurse comfortably in various positions:** Lying down or sitting with baby in "cradle" or "football" hold.

_____ **Baby is properly positioned when nursing:** Baby's head and shoulders are supported and in a straight line with his body. The baby's head is level with the breast and the baby is turned toward mom so that he can see mom with his top eye.

_____ **You feel comfortable assisting baby to latch-on:** You support your breast with one hand while using opposite arm to bring the baby up from underneath the breast. The baby's head should tilt back slightly, mouth opening wide, and his chin and lower jaw should reach the breast first.

_____ **Baby latches on well:** Takes all of nipple and about one-half to one inch of the areola into his mouth. More of the lower portion of the areola is in the baby's mouth than the upper portion. Chin and cheeks are touching the breast.

_____ **You know you are making milk:** In the first week, you may experience uterine cramping each time you nurse; you may get a sleepy feeling; you may notice tingling, pressure, or fullness in the breasts.

_____ **Baby is getting milk:** After a few short fast sucks, you notice a change in pattern to a slow, rhythmic suck-swallow. You can hear the swallow, which sounds like a sigh. When you stop nursing, you can see milk in his mouth and he may spit up some milk when he burps.

_____ **Baby is satisfied:** Your baby is relaxed at the end of the feeding. He may release the breast spontaneously, or he may drift off to sleep.

_____ **Baby is gaining weight.**

_____ **Mother is comfortable after nursing:** After the mature milk comes in, your breasts feel soft and comfortable when your baby finishes nursing. You have no lumps or engorgement.

_____ **Nipple is rounded (not pinched) when baby comes off the breast.**

_____ **Baby nurses at least 8 to 12 times each 24 hours (about every 1½ to 3 hours).**

_____ **Baby has 1 or 2 wet diapers the first day and gradually increases to at least 6 to 8 heavy wet diapers by the end of week one.**

_____ **Baby has 1 or 2 bowel movements the first day and gradually increases to 4 or more per day as the mature milk comes in:** The color changes from sticky green-black to a loose, yellow curd-like stool by the end of the first week.

Note: By about 4 weeks, bowel movements may continue as frequently as every feeding or may decrease to large amounts only once a week.

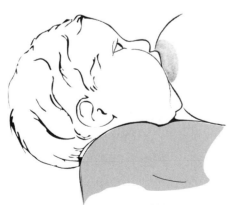

Correct Latch

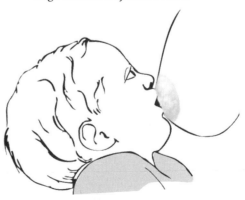

Incorrect Latch

Postpartum

People tell you how tired you'll be, but they don't tell you…that you'll be able to survive without much sleep because the simple act of looking at your baby is stirring, gratifying, energizing.

Carol Weston

The Postpartum Period

The first few hours after your baby's birth are sometimes called the fourth stage of labor. Your body begins to adjust to your new, nonpregnant state. After the placenta separates from the uterus, the uterus must contract firmly to prevent too much bleeding. The nurse will massage your *fundus* (top of the uterus) to help it contract. It should feel like a firm grapefruit at about the level of your navel. While she massages, do slow breathing to relax if it hurts. She will also check the amount of lochia (vaginal bleeding), and check your pulse and blood pressure. This will be done frequently during the first couple of hours after birth. If you have an episiotomy, an ice pack may be put on it to reduce swelling.

Most newborns are awake and alert for the first hour after birth. Keeping your baby skin-to-skin on your chest from immediately after birth through the first nursing is the best way to get breastfeeding off to a good start. Most women stay in the hospital or birth center no more than 48 hours after birth. Limit your visitors, so you can use this short time to learn to care for your baby and to have uninterrupted baby-time for breastfeeding. Take advantage of the classes offered or of personal help from your nurse. Rooming in with your baby will help you gain confidence. Before going home, ask your caregiver if you need to limit any activities such as driving, lifting, climbing stairs, sex, or exercise. This advice may vary, depending upon your individual circumstances and birth experience. Even if everything feels wonderful, remember to take it easy and not over-do when you get home.

Physical Changes

Whether you've had a vaginal or cesarean birth, your body needs time to recover. You will experience many changes as your body returns to its usual state from the physical stress of pregnancy.

- Lochia

    Immediately after birth, the vaginal discharge is bright red and heavy. It should lighten in color and amount each day until the color becomes clear. Then it will stop altogether. Although most moms will have this discharge for about four to six weeks, any *bright red* bleeding after the tenth day should be reported to your health care provider.

- Milk

    Between three and five days after birth, mom's milk supply will come in. If you nurse your baby soon after birth and frequently from the start, your breasts may not become *engorged*. But if they do feel swollen, hard, or painful, heat packs or warm water from a shower will help. Nurse your baby often to relieve the pressure.

- Uterus

    The uterus takes about six weeks to shrink to its normal pear-size shape. You may feel mild contractions as this happens. If you have given birth before these cramps may be more painful. While this is normal, if it becomes too uncomfortable, ask your health care provider to recommend an over-the-counter pain remedy.

- Sex

    You can usually start having sex after six weeks, or once vaginal flow has stopped. Both partners must feel up to it though! It may take a little time for the new mother to feel interested in sex again, especially if she had an episiotomy. If vaginal dryness is a problem, a lubricant such as K-Y jelly will help.

- Exercise

    Mom should continue to do Kegel exercises for the pelvic floor muscles. This can improve bladder control and increase awareness and pleasure during sex. Begin these soon after birth. Find a routine time to do this and do it all your life. It may help prevent problems with incontinence (leaking urine) in later years. (See page 18.) Strenuous physical exercise should not begin until after six weeks or so after birth. However, walking and mild postpartum exercises may be done as soon as you feel it is right.

Possible Physical Discomforts and Suggestions

Discomfort	Suggestions
Afterbirth contractions *Normal to feel while breastfeeding. More intense for multigravid mothers*	• Do slow breathing. • Use relaxation techniques—release all muscle groups. • Request medication for pain relief.
Difficulty urinating	• Drink lots of liquids. • Run water in sink while you try to urinate. • Pour warm water over perineum as you try to urinate. • Do Kegel exercise.
Fear of having first bowel movement	• Talk with doctor or midwife about stool softener. • Drink lots of fluids. • Eat foods high in bulk – whole grains, bran, raw vegetables, fresh and dried fruits. • Request suppository, laxative, or enema if needed.
Hemorrhoids	• Keep bowel movements as soft as possible. • Apply topical anesthetics. • Use "Tucks" (witch hazel compresses). • Kegel to promote circulation. • Discuss other medications with caregiver.
Pain from repair of episiotomy	• Apply ice pack first 12 to 24 hours. • Take warm sitz baths or tub baths. • Kegel to promote circulation. • Apply topical anesthetics (sprays or foams). • Use "Tucks" (witch hazel compresses). • Request analgesics (tell doctor if you are breastfeeding).
Breast discomforts	• See page 66.

Call your doctor or midwife if:

- your vaginal discharge (lochia)
    - is too heavy (filling one pad or more per hour)
    - turns bright red instead of dark red to brown
    - changes to foul smelling odor
    - contains blood clots larger than a golf ball
- you have pain when you urinate
- you experience cramping in legs, arms, chest, or abdomen
- your breast(s) develop painful lump(s), reddened areas or streaks, or feel hot and tender
- your abdominal incision begins to separate, develops drainage or red streaks, or if pain increases
- you are unable to have a bowel movement
- your breathing becomes difficult
- you develop a fever over 100.5°
- you have blurred vision
- you have severe headaches
- "postpartum blues" last past 2 weeks

Postpartum Emotions

The emotions that sometimes surface after birth can be a challenge. Many women have some depression or "postpartum blues" following birth. These "baby blues" are probably a combination of many factors including hormonal changes, physical discomforts, and fatigue. Some women feel let down if birth didn't go as they had hoped. Others are disappointed by not immediately regaining their pre-pregnant shape. Both parents may have anxiety about taking total responsibility for an infant. Mom may not adjust well to staying home with the baby, feeling bored or lonely. Or she may worry about returning to work if she wants to stay home. It is often difficult to balance the needs of a baby with those of other family members. Sometimes it seems that there are not enough hours in the day to get everything done. Other times it seems there are too many hours without adult companionship and help with the baby.

These "blue" feelings can last days for some women, weeks for others. The most important thing to remember about this period is that it is normal to have negative and "blue" feelings from time to time. Know that it will get better. Usually by 6 to 8 weeks postpartum, your strength returns, your family develops new routines, which include the needs of the baby. Also at this time, the baby usually starts smiling, so it all seems worthwhile. To help you with those first trying weeks, here are some suggestions from other new moms:

- Room-in at the hospital. Research shows that mothers who room-in have fewer and/or shorter periods of baby blues.

- Let your emotions out! If you feel like crying, go ahead and cry. Share your feelings with your partner. He may be experiencing many of the same feelings.

- Be a superMOM! But don't try to be Superwoman. Housework, social commitments, volunteer, and work-related activities should all take a backseat to becoming a mom. Take care of yourself as you recover, bond with your baby, get breastfeeding off to a good start, and enjoy your new family.

- Wear pajamas all day if it makes you comfortable! If you aren't dressed, you'll be more likely to go back to bed when the baby naps and perhaps visitors will stay a shorter time.

- Plan to nap daily for the first six weeks, especially if you are nursing.

- Get help with the housework and cooking. If a friend asks what she can do to help, tell her to bring a meal. If you are planning to use cloth diapers, use a diaper service or disposable diapers for the first few weeks.

- Realize that almost all babies have their days and nights mixed up at first and that almost all babies cry much more than you expect. It's okay to have occasional sad feelings and to wonder why you ever wanted to do this. Talking with friends who have young children or getting to know others from your childbirth class can be comforting. It is helpful to know that they have had similar joys and frustrations.

Seventy to eighty percent of women have the "baby blues," with feelings of worry, crying, sadness, sleep problems, mood swings, and fatigue. When these "baby blues" last longer than a month, or disrupt daily life, health professionals call this "postpartum depression." If you have more bad feelings than good feelings after birth, find a peer support group or professional help.

Ann Dunnewold, Ph.D.

Postpartum Depression

Warning symptoms that require professional help are:

- Worry, guilt, or crying that interferes with daily activities;

- Trouble sleeping, or changes in eating habits;

- Feeling like the baby dislikes you;

- Scary or bizarre thoughts that come "out of the blue," especially about harm to the baby;

- Panic attacks with powerful anxiety, fear, rapid breathing and heart rate; feeling that you are dying;

- Feeling agitated or speeded up;

- Seeing or hearing things that others do not see or hear.

If you or someone you know has these symptoms, it is important to talk to a psychologist or physician who understands pregnancy and postpartum emotional adjustment.

For the New Father

With the birth of your child, you may experience many strong emotions—pride, relief that mother and baby are fine, and a realization that lifelong responsibilities have begun.

Returning home to a new routine of diaper changes, sleepless nights, emotional ups and downs, well-meaning visitors, and a crying baby may seem to be too much. Men experience the "baby blues" too. Be aware of signs of depression in yourself as well as in mom. While you are proud of mom and fascinated with your new heir, you may grow impatient with takeout meals (or preparing your own), interrupted sleep, a less than tidy home, and having to share your wife's affection with your child. You want to offer emotional support to her, but you need emotional support too. You may wonder why you ever wanted to become a father!

To ease this change into fatherhood, it helps if you learn to take care of the baby right along with mom. Learning together and sharing feelings helps you understand one another's frustrations and joys. Just as you have shared the birth of your baby and gained a new appreciation for her, now you will share in parenting your child. Fathers have a unique way of interacting with their babies that is different from the ways that mothers interact. Babies learn from the different skills and love of both parents.

Although you have a new role as a parent, it is still important to remember your needs as a couple. Make time for each other. Love, understanding, and communication are essential. Being a parent is a lifelong team effort which produces many frustrations, but many more rewards.

Resuming Your Sexual Relationship

Like pregnancy, the postpartum period can be a stressful time in a couple's sexual relationship. In fact, many wonder if sex will ever be like it was before the baby. A couple may worry that it will be painful. If she had an episiotomy, she may be afraid that it will hurt the stitches. She may find that her vagina is so dry that sex is uncomfortable. The postpartum period is a time when both parents may be so very tired that they have no energy for romance. Newborns are emotionally demanding and need much physical touch. Some women who share this closeness with their baby all day want "their own space" when the baby is finally asleep in the evening. They may not want any more physical contact with anyone because they are drained by the baby's needs.

Bearing in mind all these concerns, it is also true that this is one of the times in a couple's relationship when a satisfying sex life can be most important. The new mother often feels "fat" and unattractive and needs to know that her mate still finds her sexually attractive. Your own intimate relationship and love for each other won't be changed by your new role as parents. Until both feel ready for more, just kissing and cuddling can be a boost to a relationship.

Suggestions that other couples have found helpful:

- Set aside a special time for sexual relations. It may be when someone else has the baby or when the baby has just been fed and you think he will sleep for a while. Take advantage of quiet mornings and afternoons when you both are more rested.

- You will ovulate and therefore may become pregnant before your first period returns. For information on family planning, consult your health care provider.

- Talk to each other – share your needs, desires, and feelings!

Observations of a Pediatrician

During the nine months or so when a woman is pregnant, she may develop motherly feelings toward her unborn baby. She may call it by a pet name and even think it has a certain personality. When the baby is born, she may feel like this is someone she already knows.

Dad, on the other hand, may greet the "little stranger" with much less sense of recognition. In fact, it may be several weeks before he thinks of the baby as a real person, with a personality all its own.

If the parents are expecting a smiling "bundle of joy," they may be in for a surprise. The baby may be coated with a white cream called *vernix*. A newborn will be wet with amniotic fluid, and occasionally blood or meconium (from the lining of the bowel). Until the baby breathes or cries, the skin is more blue to purple than it is white, brown, or black. This may worry parents if they don't know to expect it. When the baby breathes, the skin becomes a more normal color. Even then, the hands and feet may remain bluish for a while. Molding of the head allows the baby to fit through the birth canal more easily. Even a cone-shaped head at birth returns to a "normal" shape within a few days.

When first born, babies must be kept warm to hold body heat. After all, they are coming suddenly from a cozy place that has provided food, waste disposal, protection from bumps, and a finely controlled temperature. So when the birth attendant bundles mom and baby together skin-to-skin, or places the baby in an infant warmer, it is to allow gradual adjustment of the body temperature to the outside environment.

Within a few days after birth, many babies turn a yellowish color. You may have heard of it as "jaundice," a word which means yellow. This is often perfectly natural—so-called "normal" or "physiologic" jaundice. However, it may also indicate a problem, so you should check with your doctor to be sure. The yellow color moves down the body from head to trunk as the bilirubin increases. A blood test for bilirubin level may be needed. If the results are too high, your doctor may recommend treating with lights (phototherapy), either at the hospital or at home.

For most all babies, the best food is human breastmilk. Breastmilk may be expressed and frozen for later feeding. This is a way for dad to feed the baby from time to time, and will give mom a needed several hours of solid sleep, or a night out. Families with a strong history of allergies should discuss the risks of prepared formula with the baby's doctor before using it.

For valuable information in an entertaining style, read *Heading Home with Your Newborn*, written by Drs. Laura Jana and Jennifer Shu, published by the American Academy of Pediatrics.

Answers to some frequently-asked questions are:

- The "soft spot" on the baby's head is normal, and needs no special protection.
- Keep the baby's umbilical cord clean and dry to avoid infection.
- Bowel movements may occur several times a day, whenever the baby eats, or they may be several days apart after 4 weeks of age, and still be normal.
- There are reasons to circumcise and reasons not to do it. You should talk it over with your doctor.

Don't push the panic button…but it's time to call your doctor

…when your baby, who has been feeding well, loses interest in eating for a couple of feedings in a row;

…when your baby doesn't gain weight;

…when the area around the umbilical cord stump looks red, swollen, and angry;

…when there is blood or mucus in the bowel movements;

…when the baby is lethargic, or does not move about, even though awake;

…if the baby becomes jaundiced(yellow);

…when the baby feels either too hot or too cool to the touch, despite a normal room temperature and appropriate clothing or coverings; or

…when either mom or dad is worried that something may be wrong with the baby's health.

Gordon Green, M.D.

Life with Baby

What to expect

Most babies will sleep less or cry more than new parents expect. The *average* newborn sleeps 13 to 17 hours a day, and may cry one to four hours a day. That means that up to half the time baby is awake he may be crying. And that can be normal! The *very quiet* or *very active* infant sleeps or cries less than or more than the *average* baby. The only way a baby knows to call you is to cry. Crying can mean a baby is hungry, tired, hurting, too hot or too cold, or just needs a diaper changed. It may be the way your baby tells you of an emotional need to be held and protected or just to be sociable. A baby may cry when lonely or bored or after too much stimulation and play. As you get to know your baby, you will learn the difference between a sudden piercing cry of pain, the whiny continuous cry of fatigue, and the stop-and-start cry of hunger. If crying stops when you pick up your baby, it may be that he or she just needs your love and attention. Most experts today believe that it is important to respond to babies' cries, to meet both their physical and emotional needs. Babies must learn to trust. By answering cries, you help your baby establish trust with the world. You won't spoil a baby by meeting needs for cuddling and socializing. Answering cries or the cues that precede the cries (such as sucking at fists when getting hungry) teaches respect and security.

Temperament

Like each labor and birth experience, each baby is unique. Even in the womb, one mother may notice that her baby moves about vigorously at any hour of the day or night. Another mother describes more gentle movements in a regular pattern. When born, some babies are calm and quiet much of the time. When awake they may lie peacefully, entertaining themselves and moving with slow, smooth movements. Some have such a quiet intensity about them that they may even appear to be depressed. Other babies are very demanding. They want to be held and rocked seemingly all the time. Their movements are thrusting and vigorous, and their cries are long and loud. Yet others who want constant attention are bubbly and happy when they get it. At first, a quiet baby may appear to be unresponsive or an active baby uncontrollable, but you will soon learn to understand and accept the temperament and activity of your child as normal for him or her.

It is wise to listen politely to the advice of friends and family. Then trust your own instincts of how to care for *your* child. What works for others may or may not work for you. The inborn temperament of each family member contributes to the dynamics within a new family.

Quiet Baby	Average Baby	Active Baby
Cries rarely		. . . . Cries frequently, loud, and long
Sleeps much of the time		. . . . Sleeps in short periods
Lies quietly, wide-eyed		. . . . Wants attention when awake
Moves gently and slowly		. . . . Moves with vigorous thrusts and kicks
Mouths and sucks fists gently		. . . . Sucks vigorously
Enjoys bath, changing diapers		. . . . . . Cries/kicks through baths and diaper changes
Responds positively to holding, gentle rocking		. . . . . . Responds to vigorous pats, rocking, bouncing
Protests very little		. . . . Protests often
Distracted from feeding by noise or object		. . . . Nurses vigorously through distractions

Chart adapted from *Infants and Mothers* by T. Berry Brazelton, MD

States of Activity

Immediately after birth and for about ten percent of the time during the first week of life, most babies are in the **quiet alert state**. This is the perfect time to get to know your baby. They are still, but their eyes look for human faces and respond to your familiar voices. They show their natural curiosity.

After a short period in the quiet alert state, most babies will begin to move their arms and legs and enter the **active alert state**. Now baby is more easily distracted and focuses less on you. This state comes just before crying or drowsiness. You may be able to calm him, and head off the **crying state**, by putting him in a front pack or sling. Babies are often soothed by the warmth of being close to you, the sound of your heartbeat, and the movement as you walk. While some babies are content being carried for hours, others need to change activity often. A rocking chair or a swing may calm a fussy baby. Swinging, rocking, or feeding a baby may make him **drowsy**, then he will fall asleep. Most babies alternate between **quiet sleep** and **active sleep** about every thirty minutes. Some babies will nurse well if they are picked up as they begin to awaken from active sleep and fed while still calm. Others need to fully awaken to feed so they don't return to a sleep state before they have had enough to eat. You will soon learn which is better for your baby. When he returns to the quiet alert state, take advantage of this chance to play with your baby.

Quiet Alert	Active Alert	Crying
Little to no movement	Frequent episodes of movement	Vigorous movement
Watch and listen attentively	Make small sounds	Communicate need
Eyes wide open and bright	Eyes open, looking around	Eyes open or tightly closed

Drowsiness	Active Sleep	Quiet Sleep
Small movements; smiles, frowns, sucks	Slight movements: smiles, frowns, sucks	Body still
Waking or falling asleep	Breaths irregular and faster	Breaths regular
Eyes dull; no focus; eyes may roll upward	Eyes may flutter or move under lids	Eyelids closed and still

States of consciousness as described by Marshall and Phyllis Klaus in *Your Amazing Newborn*

Playing With Your Newborn

Newborns enjoy the sight of a rattle, and stare in wonder at objects hanging above them while lying on a play mat or under a mobile. But their favorite thing to look at is you! Hold and talk to your baby face-to-face. Let him see you, smell you, feel your warmth, and hear your voice. Parents often naturally change their voice when talking to a baby. Newborns react to high-pitched sounds before the lower ones. During the first month, try the following "games."

Web It!

- ❧ Talk or read, varying the pitch of your voice.
- ❧ Sing. (Babies don't care if you can't sing on key!)
- ❧ Exaggerate expressions with your face. Smile, frown, open mouth in surprise.
- ❧ Stick your tongue out and in slowly and see if baby repeats your action.
- ❧ Stroke, massage your baby with gentle pressure from chest to fingers; chest to toes; head to toes.
- ❧ Straighten, then bend baby's arms at the elbow, legs at the knee in slow, gentle exercise.

- Let baby grasp your thumbs while lying on his back. Gently help him stretch his arms over his head, then down by his side. At first, do arms together, then alternate with one arm up while other is down.
- Gently pump baby's legs, as riding a bicycle.
- Guide baby's hands to touch your face.
- Kiss and blow on baby's hands, feet, tummy.
- Shake a rattle, bell, keys, or a brightly colored ball about a foot from baby's face to let him "track" or follow the shape and sound as you slowly move it.
- As you carry your baby, talk about the smells, sights, and sounds that you notice.
- Look in a mirror together. Point to Mama, Daddy, Baby (using baby's name).
- Talk to your baby as you bathe him, change his diapers, dress him. Name the things you use and tell him what you are doing.
- Play music and dance with your baby.

As your baby grows and experiences the world, you will see many rewards for your efforts. Take time to play.

Soothing Techniques

All babies have fussy periods throughout the day. You'll learn from your baby's cues whether he or she needs more or less activity. Different techniques work for different babies. Here are a few that work for most:

- Babies love movement. Rocking, walking, or swaying settles most fussy babies. Holding your baby while gently bouncing on a birth ball may soothe him.
- Most babies love being carried in a sling or pack. Like in the womb, they can hear your heartbeat and feel the warmth of your body.
- Because babies have been snug in the womb, most enjoy being tightly swaddled.
- Babies love to snuggle with dad and sleep on his chest.
- Sometimes mimicking the "white noise" babies heard in the womb settles them down. A fan, clothes dryer, sound machine, or your own "shushing" sounds might comfort them.
- Some babies prefer to be carried over your forearm, which puts added pressure on the tummy.
- Some babies will enjoy the motion of a swing, a glider, or a bouncy seat.

Web It!

Massage

Studies with premature infants who receive daily massages show they have better weight gain and less stress while in the hospital nursery. They startle less, breathe better, and don't clench their fists as much. They are awake and active longer, but they fall asleep more quickly and sleep more soundly, with better sleep patterns. Massage also improves their overall movement and flexibility. These benefits extend to the full-term baby as well. Choose a place to do the massage where it is warm enough for the baby to be comfortable without clothes. Use a baby lotion or oil to help your hands slide easily yet firmly over each muscle group you massage.

Sleeping

Most babies sleep a lot the first day or two after birth. But that doesn't last. After that, you can pretty well count on getting little sleep at night. No matter how many books offer a solution to new-parent fatigue, there is no easy answer. Infants don't really have "sleep problems," they just don't always sleep when we want them to! Infants have a biological need to be fed; they awaken every few hours for food because they are hungry. Breastmilk is quickly digested in small stomachs, so breastfed babies frequently wake up to eat during the night, for several months. Your baby might sleep longer stretches by three or four months, or it might take them much longer before they can sleep through the night without a feeding.

According to the American Academy of Pediatrics, the safest position for most babies while sleeping is on their backs. The research shows that babies sleeping on their tummies are at a greater risk for Sudden Infant Death Syndrome (SIDS). Someone is going to tell you that babies have always slept on their tummies and been fine. Others might tell you that babies sleep better on their tummies and don't awaken themselves quite as often. The "Back-to-Sleep" campaign was proposed after research showed that babies who slept on their tummies did sleep deeper. Perhaps a few babies slept so deeply that they did not always continue to breathe.

Another possible explanation for the success of the "Back-to-Sleep" campaign is that babies re-breathe too much of their own carbon dioxide when sleeping on their tummies. A researcher, Dr. James McKenna, found that babies worldwide normally sleep on their backs, right next to their breastfeeding mother in her bed. And the rest of the world doesn't have the problem with SIDS that we do in the United States. Even if the infant is in a bassinet within a few feet of mom's and dad's bed, brain wave patterns are better than when the baby is in another room. Dr. McKenna attributes the difference to the infant's subconsciously hearing the parent's breathing and trying to mimic it.

If you practice "sleep sharing" (in bed with your baby), be sure to do it safely. The bed should have a firm mattress. Avoid soft bedding and blankets by dressing the baby warmly. The baby should be placed on her back. Beware of headboards or footboards that the baby could fall between. Never sleep with a baby if you've been drinking or using drugs.

There are several other things you can do to decrease your infants' risk of SIDS. Breastfeeding in itself is protective. Do not use fluffy comforters or pillows in cribs. Be sure the crib mattress fits tightly with no more than two-fingers' width between the side of the crib and the edge of the crib mattress. Do not allow anyone to smoke around your baby. The infant breathes in even the second-hand smoke on a smoker's clothing when held in his or her arms. Any exposure to cigarette smoke should be avoided.

Your doctor will tell you if there is a reason that your baby should not sleep on his back. Once babies begin to roll around on their own, they will sleep in the position they find comfortable, and that is fine. But until that time, most babies should be put on their back to sleep. To prevent the backs of your babies' heads from becoming "flat" from sleeping on their backs, be sure to give your babies plenty of "tummy time" when they're awake.

Feeding

Find a comfortable place to feed your baby. Keep water and pillows nearby for your comfort. Reading material, a portable phone, and the TV remote are also nice to have within reach. If you are out of bed to feed the baby at night, have a dim light in the room that you use. A small stool for propping your feet provides support to your lower back if using a rocker or glider. Some moms enjoy using a nursing pillow, but make sure it puts the baby in the right position rather than being in the way.

Diapering

You will soon master the challenge of putting a tiny diaper on your baby below the umbilical cord stump, without its falling off! This is no easy task. But since you will usually change diapers with each feeding, you will get lots of practice. Be sure to wash or sanitize your hands after every diaper change, so you don't spread germs. If you have a baby boy and you get sprayed (as you surely will), remember that urine is sterile! Then remember to cover the penis when the diaper is off and to point his penis downward when you put the clean diaper on him.

A changing station on a bathroom countertop is handy. A changing-table pad or thick towel works well here. Your baby will soon enjoy watching the activity in the mirror over the counter. Also pack a diaper bag with a waterproof changing pad, diapers, wipes, diaper rash ointment, a blanket, a change of clothes, and bags for wet things. This can be used on outings, or can "travel" around the house.

To clean baby's bottom, commercial baby wipes are handy, especially away from home. It is possible (but rare) for a baby's skin to be sensitive to them. Baby washcloths, disposable diaper liners, or cotton pads work just as well and cost less. This is easy if the changing station is by the bathroom sink for water. On baby girls, wipe from front to back with a clean area of your wipe, so bacteria from a bowel movement is not carried to the vagina. Gently clean a baby boy's penis, but do not pull back the foreskin more than it naturally goes. If he has been circumcised, the head of the penis will look purple-red and swollen in the first week. Use Vasoline, Bacitracin, or K-Y jelly on the wound until it has healed, so it won't stick to the diaper.

It is sometimes difficult to tell if a disposable diaper is wet, yet it is important to know that a baby is peeing enough. In the first week, you might put a tissue in the diaper so you can tell if even a little wetness is there. The Internet will lead you to information on the cloth vs. disposable diaper debate if you have questions. Expect to use about 10 diapers a day after the first couple of weeks.

Bathing

Swaddle-bathing works well for newborns. Wash one area of the baby's body at a time, keeping the rest of the body wrapped warmly and securely in a towel. Some health care providers recommend sponge baths until the cord falls off. Others suggest that tub baths are fine from the start. However you choose, babies only need to be washed with baby wash (soap) every few days. Do wash the baby's face and neck area with clear water every day, and clean and dry the diaper area well with every change.

Prepare the bathing area with all the supplies needed, including clean diapers and clothes. Run warm, not hot, water into a sink or baby bathtub in a room with no drafts. Remember, never take your eyes or hand off your baby for even one second when he is in the tub.

As time goes by, bath time becomes the highlight of the day. However, it is not always that way at first!

Cord Care

Usually the cord falls off by two weeks after birth, sometimes sooner, sometimes later. Most pediatricians recommend the cord be left alone until it falls off. Some doctors recommend putting alcohol on the cord to help it dry out, but others say to leave it alone. Notify your doctor if red streaks appear around the cord or if it oozes.

On the Go with Baby

The most important piece of baby equipment you will buy will be a federally-approved car safety seat. Infants are required to ride in a rear-facing car seat or car bed, depending on their weight when they leave the hospital. The back seat is the safest place for babies. Proper installation is critical. Many infant car seats come with a detachable base that stays strapped into the car when the carrier part is removed. Be sure the carrier always snaps firmly into place before driving. Some hospitals, police, and fire stations offer car seat safety inspections. Use your car seat for traveling in the car, but don't leave your baby in one for longer than necessary. When you arrive at your destination, use your stroller, sling, or pack so your baby doesn't stay in the same position for too long a time. "Wearing" your baby in a sling or infant carrier provides the baby with your warmth and in some positions, the sounds of your heartbeat and breathing.

Car seats must be purchased new or from someone you know. If used, be sure that it has never been in a car during an accident. Even a "mild" crash at 30 mph can make a car seat unsafe because of an invisible hairline crack. Call the Auto Safety Hot Line at 888-327-4236 to be sure the model you choose has not been recalled.

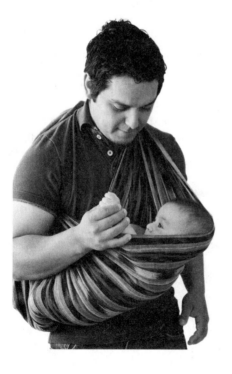

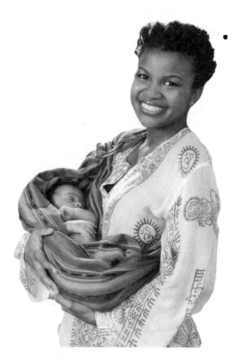

Baby Gear

Dress babies according to the temperature. If it isn't cold, they don't need to be wrapped in heavy blankets! Many babies cry because they are too hot or too cold. Babies quickly outgrow their clothes. How many outfits you need depends on how often you plan to do laundry. It is a rare day that a baby will wear only one outfit, due to spit-up and leaks. Changing bibs sometimes prevents changing an outfit. Wash only a few of each type clothing you get, to see which you like to use. Extra items with tags left on could then be exchanged if you don't use them. What one mother may tell you she used every day may not work for you at all. See the chart below for suggestions on various items you may use.

Basic Layette and Bedding Needs	Basic Baby Equipment	Medications and Infant Care
• Crib or bassinet	NECESSARY:	• Thermometer
• Diapers, cloth – 3 dozen	• Infant car seat	• Lubricant for thermometer
• Diapers, disposable – 300 the first month	HELPFUL:	• Re-hydrating fluid such as Pedialyte®
• Burp cloths	• Bathtub or bath sling	• Liquid acetaminophen such as Tylenol®
• Bibs	• Head support for carseat	• Medicine syringe or dropper
• Baby washcloths	• Diaper pail	• Liquid baby wash
• Baby hooded towel	• Changing area	• Baby lotion
• "Onesies" / undershirts	• Baby carrier or sling	• Diaper rash ointment
• Gowns / sleepers	• Stroller	• Baby nail-clippers/emery board
• Booties	• Rocker	• Infant saline drops
• Crib sheets	• Swing, bouncy seats	• Q-tips®
• Waterproof crib pads	• Nursing pillow	• Bulb syringe
• Waterproof lap pads	• Breast pump	• Baby detergent for laundry
• Baby hats	• Cordless phone	• Soft brush for lightly scrubbing hair while shampooing, to prevent cradle cap
• Swaddle blankets	• Chair with footstool	
• Heavier blankets	• Baby monitor	
• Sweater as needed for climate or season	• Small penlight to check on babies at night	

Safety

Although many of the following ideas won't apply until your baby becomes mobile, that time will sneak up on you. Here's a list for you to use over the next year to get ready for that day.

Post the number for the Poison Control Center near your phone.

What types of live plants do you have in your home? Know their names and contact the Poison Control Center to find out if they are safe or poisonous.

Tie up your mini-blind cords to prevent possible strangulation.

Block off all electrical outlets with inserts or furniture to prevent electric shock.

Cushion the brick around your fireplace hearth if it is an area that will be available to your baby; remove pokers and other fireplace equipment.

Make sure that all cribs and baby furniture or toys that could be chewed on have only lead-free paint.

Install gates over stairway entrances and other hazardous areas of your house.

Install cabinet locks for all cabinets that contain potentially harmful products. (The most effective cabinet locks are Tot-Loks®, a magnetic lock that won't allow the cabinet to be opened without the special magnet the parents keep up high.) The cheapest and most effective prevention is to remove harmful products from low cabinets. Keep them higher than a toddler can reach.

Make sure furniture can't be tipped over when your baby starts pulling up. Secure chests of drawers to the wall.

Remove all grocery store plastic bags and the like from areas that toddlers can reach.

Install a toilet lid lock, or get into the habit of keeping the bathroom doors shut at all times.

Remove flowing tablecloths that could be a hazard when your baby starts pulling up.

Plan a fire safety escape route.

Install fire alarms and carbon monoxide sensors.

Cushion sharp edges of coffee tables and furniture.

Adjust the thermostat on your water heater so the hot water can't come out above 120°, to prevent scaldings.

Buy a thermometer or tub toy to check the baby's bath water. About 85° is recommended for a newborn's bath temperature.

Check small toys for choking hazards by using the toilet paper roll test. If the toy can fit into a toilet paper roll, it can be swallowed, and possibly could block a baby's airway.

Plan to use stationary toys like Exersaucers® or other baby seats, rather than walkers.

Visit your local fire or police station, or hospital to be sure you have your car seat properly installed.

Remove all bedside medications, lotions, perfumes, etc. to a safe location.

Birth Stories

The birth of a baby is an everyday miracle…a deep
and permanent memory for the birthing woman and
those who love her and support her.

Penny Simkin

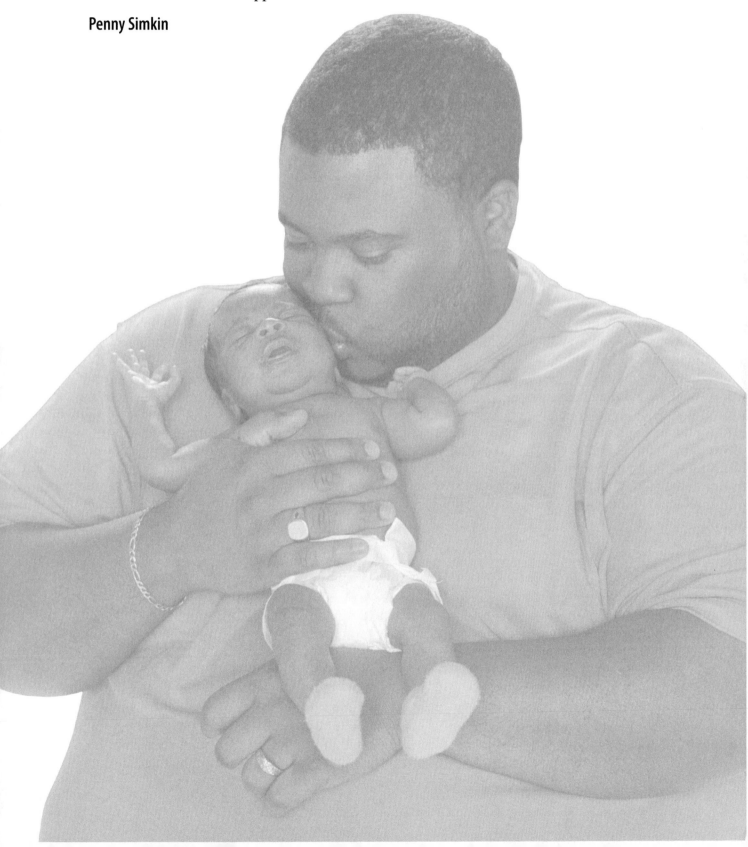

Cary's Birth Story

After waiting 32 years to have a baby, I was extremely excited when I found out I was pregnant, and a little "over eager" to soak up any information I could find on childbirth. So much so, that at 10 weeks, my husband Steve and I attended an early pregnancy class. Most everyone in the class was planning for an epidural, but I was curious about the possibility of natural childbirth. Our instructor suggested that we consider a doula, a concept we were not familiar with but one we were both very interested in.

My pregnancy was healthy and uneventful until the 30th week when we ended up with a midnight trip to the hospital with painful contractions. After discovering that the contractions were coming regularly every two minutes, I was given medication to help them stop, then sent home for 10 weeks of bedrest. This was a complete shock to us since pregnancy had gone so smoothly, but we followed our orders strictly in order to avoid a premature birth. The 10 weeks seemed to drag on with nothing to do but to read about, think about, and talk about the upcoming event and baby we so eagerly awaited. One helpful thing I did during this time was to watch the video of my sister's birth. Seeing her come through it so well, I was confident that I should be able to succeed too.

After a routine checkup at 37 weeks, my doctor was concerned that the baby might be very large and began talking about the possibility of inducing. I was not eager to do this, but at 38 weeks when he suggested using prostaglandin gel to soften my cervix, I agreed. The only effects I felt from the gel were slight cramps and the discomfort of having it inserted. At 41 weeks, and still no sign of labor, I was feeling extremely anxious and agreed to try the gel again that evening. At 6:00 the next morning, my water broke.

We arrived at the hospital at 7:30 after calling my doctor, my doula, our family, and a few friends. We had decided earlier that we wanted our family at the hospital, but the only people we planned to have in the birthing room were ourselves and our doula. At around 8:00, my doula arrived and I immediately felt calm. Her presence alone gave me a huge dose of confidence. Shortly after, I was seen by the doctor and told that if I wasn't in a regular labor pattern by noon, he wanted to induce. That was all the motivation I needed to take to the halls and walk. Steve was extremely nervous at this point and our doula sensed it and gave him some needed "time off." So I walked and walked and walked accompanied by Jeanne, stopping only to breathe through my contractions. The time spent walking and talking with her was very helpful in passing the time. Her gentle encouragement continued to boost my confidence making me think, "I can do this - I'm DOING this!" Up to this point, the contractions were only a little stronger than very hard menstrual cramps, but as noon approached, they started getting much more intense. It was around this time that my mother and sister arrived at the hospital. I hadn't expected to be so glad to see them or to be so overwhelmed with emotion when they entered the room. But when they came in, I knew that I wanted them to stay. The combination of doula, family, and spouse was perfect for me. I felt so loved and supported at all times – something I hadn't anticipated cherishing so dearly about the birth process.

I had progressed in dilation from barely a 1 to a 4 during this time. The time between noon and 3:00 was a blur of one strong contraction after another. The pain never felt too intense to handle, but I worked hard on remaining very focused on my breathing. Another helpful tool for me was music. I had tried out several relaxing CD's prior to labor and found one I was particularly fond of. I played it continuously throughout labor on my "walkman" which seemed to help me go deep inside myself during the particularly difficult contractions. I began to experience back labor and leg pain during this time and found much comfort in massage and touch that my sister and doula so freely gave.

At 3:00, I had progressed to an 8 and began feeling the urge to push, which for me was BY FAR the most difficult part of the labor process. In describing it to Steve, I said that it felt like a freight train was running through my body at full speed and I was having to hold it in. I began to have my first panicky feelings of doubt as this phase of labor wore on. If not for the continuous encouragement and sometimes rather specific instructions to "Blow!" I would have fallen apart. At around 4:45 I was given the go ahead to push and I was determined that things were going to quickly "come to a head." I pushed with every ounce of strength I had whenever I felt the urge and within 4-5 pushes, Caroline's head was crowning. The doctor was not yet in the room and everyone was surprised when on the very next push, Caroline's entire head was out. Everything and everyone seemed to be moving in slow motion. I remember the nurse yelling for the doctor while telling me not to push, but all I cared about and all I could focus on was Caroline, the little head I saw in the mirror. I was oblivious to all else. The doctor did arrive and after another push, I had a beautiful (and average-sized) baby girl lying on my chest at 5:09 p.m. I had a small tear that required a few stitches, but I wasn't phased by it after laying eyes on Caroline. She was extremely alert for several hours and my sister remarked that she seemed like an old soul – very wise, the way she gazed so intently at each of us. After the birth, I felt completely exhilarated and euphoric. I felt invincible and capable of accomplishing anything. I hadn't known fully what to expect from a natural childbirth, but it far surpassed my highest expectations and wildest dreams, and I would never want to do it any other way. These wonderful feelings came in handy and helped me not to become too discouraged when we had difficulty breastfeeding.

Caroline didn't seem interested in breastfeeding and had difficulty latching on from the very beginning. I was nervous and unsure, and hearing her shriek and arch away from me when I put her to my breast was very disheartening. I was prepared through my reading and childbirth classes that it didn't always happen perfectly right away so I wasn't completely discouraged. But it was unsettling and it began to eat away at my confidence. I felt labeled as "the one who cannot nurse" and began to feel truly discouraged when they wanted me to give her formula. My mother and sister kept encouraging me to stick with it which helped tremendously.

Our nursing problems continued for 2 weeks. The only way I could get her to take any breastmilk was to pump and feed her from a bottle. I would continue to offer her my breast and she continued to reject it. I had all but given up hope and resolved to pump "forever" in order to provide her with the benefits of breastmilk if that's all I was able to do. When magically, late one night at the two-week mark while warming a bottle, I tried again and she latched on and nursed as if it were all she had ever known. In fact, after that night, she would never take another bottle or pacifier.

I encourage all of the first time moms to believe in yourselves and your God-given abilities to give birth. Trust your gut and your instincts and surround yourselves with positive, encouraging people. Never underestimate the power of support. It made all the difference in the world for me and made Caroline's birth an experience I'll treasure forever.

Cary & Steve Odom

A Special Birth

One morning in the middle of April, I awoke and blurted out to my husband that the previous night I had gotten pregnant. He looked at me, laughed…mumbled something about a vivid imagination and totally dismissed the subject. Four weeks later, after a visit to my OB-GYN, I walked into his office and announced that the rabbit had died. From then on (at least where my pregnancy was concerned), I was convinced I was psychic. It was just a matter of patience now, after all "Madame Lorie" knew that in nine months she would be giving birth to a beautiful baby boy and have the smoothest birth ever to be recorded in medical archives.

My pregnancy was literally textbook. A little morning sickness in the second and third month, but aside from that, I was your typical radiant and happy pregnant lady. I quit my job in my fourth month…basked in my husband's attention and read everything even remotely connected with my condition and babies. From the beginning I wanted to attempt an unmedicated birth and was determined to be as well-prepared as possible. In my seventh month, Chris (my husband) and I registered for our Lamaze classes where we learned to pelvic-tilt, breathe, and Kegel the rest of my pregnancy away.

On my due date, January 8th, I was informed by my doctor that most likely I'd be about a week late. The baby was in position but had not dropped yet and by my calculations that seemed about right. So that day I went home planning to go shopping the next day for slippers to match the robe I had gotten for Christmas.

Saturday, January 9th, I awoke at 5:00 a.m. with a very strong cramping sensation in my lower abdomen. I went to the bathroom thinking it would probably stop momentarily…it did…five minutes later it returned. By 5:30, I woke Chris up and made the intelligent statement that I didn't know what was happening but whatever it was, it was happening every 5 minutes. We called the doctor, who advised us to go to the hospital.

"No, no!" I kept thinking, this isn't the way it's going to be. Where was my quiet time? I was supposed to be playing cards…watching TV…relaxing…and anyway I wasn't going to have my baby for another week. I refused to call the sensations I was experiencing "labor," and was sure they'd send me back from the hospital despite the strength of my contractions. Vanity above everything, I insisted on showering and washing my hair before leaving and, oh yes, packing my suitcase.

At 8:00 a.m. we arrived at the hospital, and by 8:05 were officially told that I was in labor. At my arrival I was 3 cm. dilated and when my doctor came in an hour later I was up to 4 cm.

Once in the hospital and convinced I was actually in labor, we really started to work. Side by side we walked up and down the corridor. The contractions were coming strong and steady – about every 3 minutes – and I really had to breathe to get through them; but we were handling it well. We couldn't help but be somewhat disappointed when at noon the doctor announced I was still at 4 cm. Around 1:30 p.m., he decided to break my water. On doing this, he observed signs of meconium, so I was connected to a fetal monitor, where the electrode is applied to the baby's scalp. Being on the monitor was uncomfortable mostly because it limited me to, at best, a semi-reclining position, but it was worth it to know that my baby was in no immediate danger. An hour later, still at 4 cm. the doctor suggested pitocin, hoping that it would get me to dilate. The pitocin was administered through an IV that was hooked up earlier. My contractions had been strong since the beginning of my labor, growing with intensity and duration by the hour. After the pitocin, however, I felt close to despair. I couldn't concentrate on my focal point and the contractions seemed to be taking over my entire body. My husband came to the rescue. He gently but firmly talked me into relaxing and breathed with me until slowly I began regaining control. At 4:30 p.m., still at 4 cm., my doctor came in and said the word I thought I'd never hear – cesarean. Chris and I had been looking forward to a totally natural birthing experience…but by this point our main concern was having a healthy baby. For some reason I was not dilating, despite having been in active labor for 10 hours, and because of the meconium, there was an added risk. All I wanted was for something to happen. By 5:00 p.m. I had been prepped, given an epidural, and wheeled into the operating room. Chris left my side only long enough to suit up. When he walked in and sat by me I looked into his eyes and smiled. A feeling of peace and confidence that we had made the right decision overcame me and from that moment on I knew everything would be fine.

Soon our little person came into the world protesting loudly the release from the womb that had reluctantly let go. Almost miraculously, the minute Chris cradled and talked to our child, the cries ceased. I felt drunk and giddy with joy…we were finally three. So at 5:46 p.m. another one of my famous predictions came true…. I had a beautiful baby. The only slight deviation was that we had to call her Jessica instead of James.

Just a few end notes. I breastfed my baby in the recovery room and we established a beautiful nursing relationship from day one. Jessica is a happy and healthy child, bringing into our lives more happiness than we thought possible. My recovery from surgery was very fast and in six weeks (thanks to nursing) I had lost 30 of the 40 lbs. I gained during pregnancy. I lost those last 10 lbs. too, but I still don't have a pair of slippers to match the robe I got for Christmas.

Lorie & Chris Roberts

The Long and Short Of It

After giving birth for the second time, I was amazed at how different two labors could be. I wouldn't trade the experience of either of them, because each brought us a baby – the most precious gift in the world.

With our first child our story began on a Tuesday, four days before our due date. I was upset when my doctor informed me that day that it would be one to two weeks before I would deliver. I decided to try to change that prediction, so for the next two nights Larry and I played tennis. Perhaps that did the trick, for at 6 a.m. on Thursday I lost my mucus plug and my contractions began.

At noon my contractions were ten minutes apart and easy to handle. By 6 p.m. they still did not require much concentration, but I was certainly aware they were there – every five to seven minutes. Larry and I decided to have supper just in case we were going to need the energy later. Although these contractions had been going on all day, I kept telling myself this was false labor—but it wasn't. From 9 p.m. to midnight, contractions came every three minutes and lasted ninety seconds. This had to be labor. We called the doctor and went to the hospital. The nurse checked me and I was only 2 centimeters dilated and 90% effaced. Oh, how disappointing! Contractions all day and only 2 cm. We decided to walk and walk and walk. A check at 4 a.m. told us the baby was posterior and I was only 3-4 cm. dilated. I was having back labor. There was pain in my back even when there were no contractions. Time was passing slowly, contractions were getting harder, and I was losing my concentration. I was given some medication to help me relax. Larry applied counterpressure to my low back and gave me lots of encouragement, though he too was exhausted. I told him I could not take any more, but he told me I could—and I did. At 7 a.m. the baby still had not turned, but I had made it to 9 cm. At full dilation, I had no urge to push, making it difficult to do so. With the support of my husband and doctor I did get the baby pushed down enough for her to be manually rotated. It then took about ten more hard pushing contractions before our 8 pound-14½ ounce daughter, Holly Rene, was born. It was a long and difficult labor, but Holly was worth it.

As Larry and I were adjusting to being parents, we found out it wouldn't be long until we were parents of two. Believe me, nursing your baby does not prevent you from getting pregnant. I was due again fourteen months after Holly's birth.

The day before this due date the doctor told me I was 2 cm. dilated and 60% effaced. He said I would probably go another week before the birth. This time I did not play tennis, but that night I did not sleep well due to some strong Braxton-Hicks contractions. By 10 a.m., I was deciding perhaps these were true contractions, so I finished the laundry, packed, and left for the doctor's office. My doctor said I was 3 cm. dilated, and 80% effaced. He gave us the choice of going home to wait or going to the hospital for him to break my bag of waters to see if labor would pick up. We opted for the latter. When my water was broken there was no immediate change in my contractions. I was 4 cm. and a minus 3 station. An hour later I was 6 cm. and a minus 1 station. Things certainly were progressing faster than last time! I began to need the breathing techniques around 3:30 when I was about 7 cm. dilated. How different than before. I had decided that this time I was going to sit up or walk as long as I possibly could in hopes this would give me that *urge* to push. During transition I was able to relax and knew all that was going on around me. This baby, too, was posterior – I guess that's the way I carry babies. My doctor had me lie on my side to help the baby turn. I then needed Larry to give some counterpressure during some of the contractions, though it was nothing like the back labor I'd had before. At 4:30, I was 8 cm. and had a small urge to push. Five minutes later I was 10 cm. and *the urge* arrived in full force. The birthing bed was made ready. It was good to be in control with gentle pushing. No episiotomy was necessary. The sensation of giving birth was marvelous once again.

Shelly & Larry Eswein

A Proud Grandma's Story

I want to share with you a love story!

Five days ago, I became the grandmother of the most precious little boy on earth! Juan Manuel arrived two weeks early, taking us all by surprise.

His birth has been the most amazing and memorable experience that I have witnessed in recent times. It can only be compared to what I felt at the births of my daughters. It has touched and changed my life forever.

It was truly a labor of love, into which my daughter surrendered, listening to her body, and trusting it completely. Even when some of those around her doubted that a natural birth would be possible, she acted with great confidence and ability, showing them otherwise. She never lost her good nature and sense of humor. After 40 hours of very hard work (two days and two nights), she triumphantly came out of this experience feeling on top of the world, more mature and womanly than I could have ever imagined. Here was this girl who dreaded shots, cried like a baby at the sight of a syringe, and made such a huge fuss about them, working beautifully through huge contractions with a persistent posterior presentation that never rotated no matter what she tried and, as you might have guessed, a bad case of back labor. She never complained about the long hours or the grueling pain. Her only concern was for her baby and her fears of ending with a cesarean or huge interventions. Fortunately, her obstetrician never gave up on her, and sat by her side waiting for nature to take its course. After being stuck for three hours at 7 cm., she was finally completely dilated within the next hour. Almost three hours of pushing later, little Juan Manuel was born facing his mother (posterior) and with his fist on his chin. He was crying even before leaving his mother's body, but when placed on his mom's belly the cries changed into suckling sounds as he licked his mother's breast and found his way to her nipple.

At that exact moment I thanked God from the bottom of my heart for the incredible miracle that I had just witnessed. There are no words to describe what I felt a few moments later when my son-in-law, tears rolling down his face, placed my grandson in my arms and he gazed straight into my eyes.

It has been a unique and wonderful privilege to have served my daughter as her doula. I feel honored and blessed for this opportunity. I have witnessed an incredible transformation in my daughter as she entered motherhood. My admiration, respect, and love for her grow indefinitely. I am sure they will be the best parents and the most loving!

Elena Carrillo
The proudest grandma in the world

A Dad's Story

I suppose it's axiomatic to describe childbirth as a surreal experience. The whole process is surreal, really—from the happy shock of conception to the first ultrasound, first heartbeat, first bulge, first kick and, finally, to the day we get to meet our baby. Certainly not your normal 9 months. A side effect of this whole process—or, perhaps more accurately, the length of the process—was that the idea of being a daddy was somehow stuck as a "future" event in my head.

So on May 28, 2008, I knew Charlie was supposed to be coming the next day, his due date, but I did not expect it to happen. I was just sure that we were going to meander through life for another week or two before labor actually began. All that changed when my wife, Jordan, made a seemingly innocuous comment about having some "cramping" before going to bed that night. I didn't recall Jordan ever complaining about cramping before, and it took my normally Neanderthal brain about 4½ seconds to conclude that I was going to be a daddy in the very near future.

An hour later, we had confirmation, as the cramping quickly became increasingly frequent contractions. Jordan had not had any pre-labor contractions, so this was our first shot at the dog-and-pony show of getting the pregnant lady to the hospital. Surprisingly, everything went just fine. I called my mom, a nurse, and she walked us through what was happening with Jordan's body and what we should be looking out for. Jordan was in some minor discomfort but handling it like a champ (it doesn't hurt that she has the pain threshold of a medieval monk). While we waited for the contractions to reach the "to-the-hospital" threshold, I took a shower and quickly packed a bag. I wouldn't really say I was nervous or concerned at this point, just focused on making sure we had what we needed to get to the hospital. Well, that's not exactly true–I was actually very nervous but able to focus on the task at hand. Then Jordan told me that her water broke. Bam, we were in the car and on the way to the hospital.

We got to the hospital sometime after midnight, and Jor was still doing great. We took some final belly pictures beside the car in the parking lot and made our way through the largely deserted labyrinth of the hospital's labor-and-delivery department. The nurses were great and quickly had Jordan resting comfortably in a private room. We were adorned with wristbands and identification tags. The midwife was en route to the hospital, and our families were making their way to our home in Houston, Texas. Jordan was going to have a natural childbirth, so our charge now was just to wait for Charlie to make his way into the world. At this point, I was hoping for a quick, painless birth and lots of smiles and patting each other on the back in the morning. I was wrong.

I was off a bit on the timing. For some reason, I had it in my head that a birth should take between 3 and 5 hours, or somewhere in that range. As apparently everybody else but me is aware, first-time births routinely take 12 or 16 hours or more. I learned this little factoid sometime in the wee hours when I sensed things were not progressing on my schedule. Worse, the real labor contractions had started to pick up in both frequency and severity. It's tough to see your wife in apparent (but not actual) distress and know that there is nothing you can do for her. Still, Jor's the champ, and she powered through with a (diminishing) smile on her face. By 3:30 a.m., the smile was gone, and the situation—from my naive eyes, at least—seemed dire. Luckily, women are equipped to deal with this stage of labor, and Jordan's own body (remember, no drugs) provided her with the painkillers she needed. She seemed to enter into a trance-like state, as if she had just exited the "happy tent" at the Woodstock music festival. Good for her.

Around 4:00 a.m., Jordan's best friend, Maggie, and my mom, Debby, arrived. Both have extensive professional experience in childbirth. I was putting on a brave face while, inwardly, I was terrified; in contrast, they were unperturbed. It is at this point that I have trouble recalling the exact events that took place. The fatigue and adrenaline took a toll on whatever part of my brain that is tasked with long-term storage. I do know that Maggie and my mom did an absolutely wonderful job with Jordan. They repeated, ad nauseam, encouraging and comforting words as they walked Jordan from the bed to the bath, and back, and to wherever else she felt comfortable for a few minutes. Later in the morning, the contractions continued their assaults, and we started getting some significant dilation. The midwife arrived to help Jordan give birth to Charlie in the room, and she, too, was wonderful. Things were starting to look up.

By 11:00 a.m., it looked like the end was in sight. Jordan was in pain (she appeared to be in death throes) but later said it wasn't nearly as bad as it looked. Everybody was tired but really happy to meet Charlie. The very end, to put it nicely, was not a thing of poetic beauty. Labor had been going on for well over 12 hours. There was sweat, there were screams, there was cutting, and there was blood. But all of that was forgotten when Charlie's head popped out and I got my first look at my son. The feeling of seeing your child for the first time is, as many have said, indescribable. If you've been there, you know. Unfortunately for me, that moment was momentarily interrupted when I noticed that Charlie was born with an extremely pointy head. He was a conehead. Another gaffe on my part, as the nurses—who apparently deal regularly with fathers who are as knowledgeable as I am—quickly told me that Charlie was fine and that his head would soon take a normal shape. It did. Charlie had some initial problems getting situated and, as a precaution, the nurses whisked him out of the room. I followed and, after about 5 minutes, was finally able to hold him for the first time.

I figured Jordan would be in a coma for at least 2 days as soon as that kid popped out. Again, I was wrong. As soon as labor was over, she became her normal, chipper self, as if the last 14-plus hours never happened. And, something I'll never forget, I don't think I've ever seen Jordan quite as happy as when I laid Charlie on her chest for the first time.

Brian Amis
For Brian, Jordan, Charlie & Tommy

At Long Last

I have a birthday story to tell. It is not a short and simple one, but it has a very happy ending. Our baby girl was due around the first of April, but she just wasn't quite ready to come then! I walked for miles that last month. I talked to her and tried just about everything anyone suggested to start my labor, but nothing worked. Finally I agreed with my doctor that if she didn't come before April 14, I would be induced. It was put on the schedule. But as it happened, my contractions began around midnight the night before, and I was well into labor by induction time that morning. When contractions were about 5 minutes apart, we went to the hospital. I was 4 cm dilated and 90% effaced! That was good news and good progress at 5 am. The morning passed with good, frequent contractions. By noon, my cervix was fully effaced, but had only gained a centimeter. The baby was high at a minus 2 station. We tried to coax her down with lots of movement. For hours, I walked and rocked and swayed and lunged. My doula rubbed my back to help me relax and kept me trying new things. I found a rhythm in labor and was willing to try anything that was suggested. Andrew held me close, and was very loving and encouraging. His support gave me strength. I rocked on hands and knees, leaning over the labor ball, and tried all sorts of positions to try to help her move. Lunch time passed, dinner time came… and passed. Finally 7:00 p.m. and only 7 cm. Three cm in 15 hours was not what we planned! The doctor thought that Pitocin might help, so that was started, along with an epidural. Labor still didn't progress quickly, but the epidural gave me relief from the contractions. The doctor determined that the baby was posterior and high, and that a cesarean may be in the future if that didn't change. I changed my positions between side and sitting, trying to help her turn. By midnight I at last reached 10 cm dilation. Now it was April 15th, taxes were due, and she wasn't out yet! But three hours later, she was heading down and was reachable with forceps. So at 3:23 am, after lots of hard pushing, Miss Caroline Rae arrived. It was a relief to everyone, including our families who had been in the waiting room a very long time!

This was not the labor of my dreams, but I did have wonderful support from family, doctor, and staff. And best of all I had a precious, healthy baby girl in my arms. You can't beat that. Still, maybe next time we will try a short version!

… And Shortly After

Two years later, I have another, very different birth story to tell. Once again I tried everything to beat an induction date. (My babies prefer 42 weeks inside!) I even added acupuncture to my list. Something worked… this time my water broke at home while my doula was visiting and my husband was coming in the door. Contractions immediately started coming hard and fast. I finished packing while on my hands and knees and talking to my doctor on the phone. Wasting no time, we dropped Caroline off with a friend and drove to the hospital in rush-hour traffic. Trying to focus and breathe wasn't easy! I couldn't believe things were moving so quickly. Catherine Belle was born just 3 hours after my first contraction with none of the procedures I had before. Now THIS was more like the labor of my dreams!

Christy & Andrew McWhorter

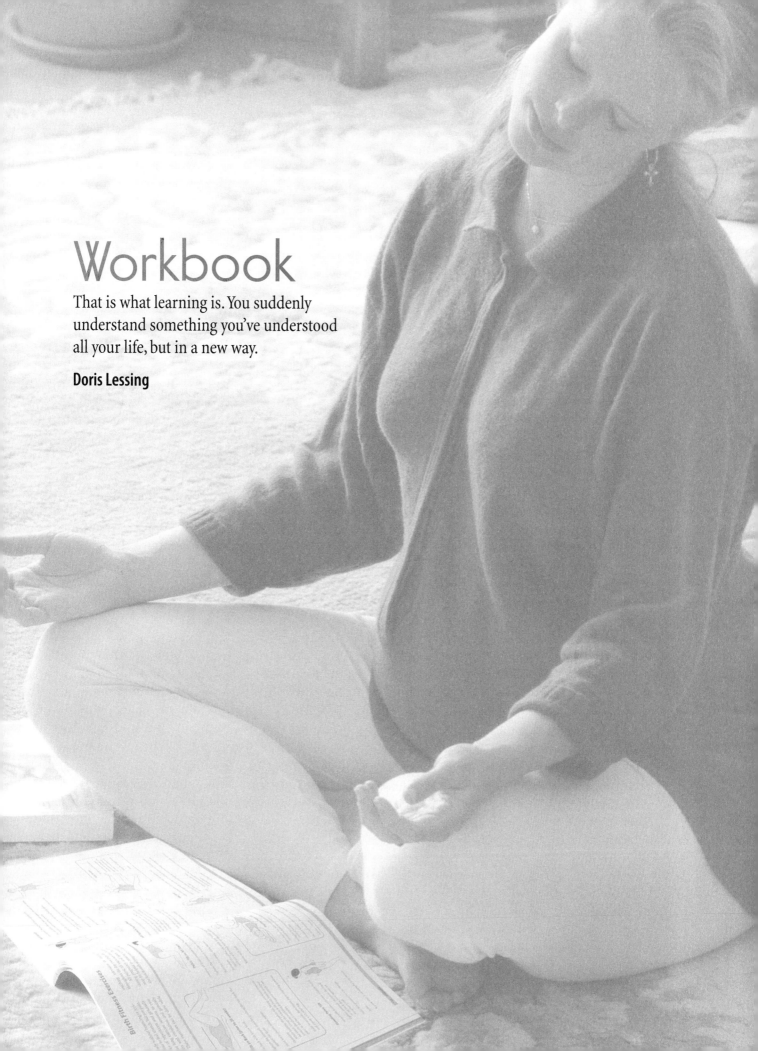

Workbook

That is what learning is. You suddenly understand something you've understood all your life, but in a new way.

Doris Lessing

Weekly Review

To get the most from this book and your childbirth classes, spend time reviewing information and practicing skills. The birth fitness exercises will make you feel better. They help circulation, relieve backache, and increase flexibility. A perfect way to end an exercise session is to "actively" relax. When you learn these stress-relieving skills, you will use them in many life situations. Focusing on your breathing will help you relax and give you more energy. Move into different positions for comfort as you try various breathing and relaxation techniques. If you practice them in pregnancy, you are more likely to listen to your body, adapt the skills, and to do what works for you in labor. Partners who practice together will find it easier to identify and release tension, and to concentrate on the familiar breathing patterns in labor. You will feel like a team prepared for birth.

Discuss your plans with each other. Use the following chart to keep track of the information covered.

		Week				
		1	2	3	4	5 and after
General	Mom and partner read *Prepared Childbirth – The Family Way*					
	Use good body mechanics – pgs. 14-15					
	Set wellness goals for pregnancy – pg. 97					
	Do *Nutrition Crossword Puzzle* – pg. 101					
	Complete the *Diet Evaluation* – pg. 103					
	Answer *How Well Do You Know Your Body?* – pg. 99					
	Complete *Pain Medication Preference Scale* – pg. 110					
	Pack your goody bag – pg. 96					
	Complete *Birth Options Chart* – pg. 111					
Exercises	Practice birth fitness exercises – pgs. 16-19					
	Do *Kegel* exercises – pg. 18					
	Try *Fun and Fast Format for Feeling Fit and Flexible* – pg. 100					
	Walk or other aerobic exercise – pg. 19					
Relaxation & Breathing	Review *Active Relaxation Techniques* – pgs. 24-26					
	Practice progressive tense/release exercise – pg. 104					
	Review touch relaxation – pg. 26					
	Complete *Relaxing Words* – pg. 105					
	Complete *Relaxing Images* – pg. 106					
	Try breathing strategies in your everyday life – pg. 43					
	Practice Rhythmic Breathing – pg. 107					
	Complete *With This Birth, I Plan to Try* – pg. 108					

What to Pack

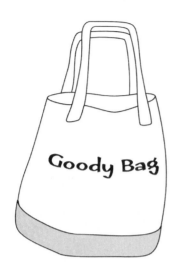

Goody Bag
For Labor

_____ This handbook

_____ Robe and slippers for walking during labor

_____ Focal point(s)

_____ iPod® or other music player

_____ Sour candy on a stick

_____ Colored washcloths

_____ Lotion or oil for massage (scented, if you like)

_____ Lip balm

_____ Mouthwash and/or toothbrush and toothpaste

_____ Deck of cards, magazine, book

_____ Nutritious snack for partner

_____ Contact lens case and eyeglasses

_____ Warm socks

_____ One or more items for back massage

_____ Vibrating pillow and/or vibrating massager

_____ List of people to call or text after the birth (including your childbirth educator)

_____ Cash for vending machine

_____ Band for long hair

_____ Fan

_____ Hand mirror to view pushing

_____ Paper and pencil

_____ Camera and/or video recorder

_____ Extra pillows with colored pillowcases

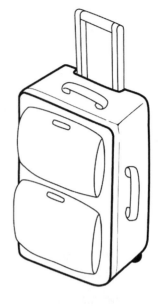

Suitcase
For Postpartum

_____ Nursing gowns or pajamas (it is nice to have hidden openings in the front)

_____ Robe

_____ Slippers

_____ Nursing bras (you will probably need a full cup size larger than you wore before you were pregnant)

_____ Nursing pads (cloth or paper)

_____ A good breastfeeding book

_____ Toilet articles

_____ Hair care items

_____ Cosmetics

_____ Going home outfit for mom–early pregnancy size

_____ Going home outfit and blanket for baby

_____ A good book

_____ Baby book (for footprints)

_____ Labor and Birth Questionnaire (page 117)

Also
For the Ride Home

_____ Infant car seat

Wellness Goals for Pregnancy

	Mom's Goals	Target Date	Progress
Nutrition			
Exercise			
Stress Management Techniques			
Other			

	Partner's Goals	Target Date	Progress
Nutrition			
Exercise			
Stress Management Techniques			
Other			

Counting Baby's Movements

Feeling your baby move or kick is very reassuring. It tells you that your baby is doing well. If there is a decrease or sudden change in movements, however, your baby needs to be checked. Some caregivers ask all pregnant women to chart "fetal movements" after 32 weeks of pregnancy. Others ask only high-risk women to do this. You may find that charting your baby's movements is fun and helps you not to worry. It gives you special time to focus on his or her activity. But some women say it makes them worry to do this. Talk to your caregiver about what is best for you. There are many ways to do this and many opinions on how many movements you should feel within a certain amount of time.

The "Count to Ten" method is a popular way to chart movements. Start when baby is awake and active. Often, a good time is after eating a meal. Count each kick, wiggle, twist, roll, or flutter as one movement. Don't count hiccups as movements. After a few kicks, the baby may fall asleep. Continue your count when the movements begin again.

When you are ready to count, place an "X" on the chart when you feel the baby move. Count each movement until you reach 10, then again mark the chart. In the example below, mom felt her baby move at 11:00 a.m. and began the count. The 10th move came at 1:00 p.m. The time it takes to count 10 movements may change from day to day, just as the baby's sleep/wake cycle changes. Call your caregiver if, over a period of several days, it is taking longer and longer to complete 10 movements.

Some caregivers ask that you call if you don't feel ten movements within a certain time limit. Ask your caregiver about his or her guidelines for you.

"Count to 10" Chart

	Week							Week							Week							Week						
	Su	M	Tu	W	Th	F	S	Su	M	Tu	W	Th	F	S	Su	M	Tu	W	Th	F	S	Su	M	Tu	W	Th	F	S
6 a.m.																												
7 a.m.																												
8 a.m.																												
9 a.m.																												
10 a.m.	X																											
11 a.m.																												
12 noon																												
1 p.m.	X																											
2 p.m.																												
3 p.m.																												
4 p.m.																												
5 p.m.																												
6 p.m.																												

(Example column marked between 11 a.m. and 12 noon.)

	Week							Week							Week							Week						
	Su	M	Tu	W	Th	F	S	Su	M	Tu	W	Th	F	S	Su	M	Tu	W	Th	F	S	Su	M	Tu	W	Th	F	S
6 a.m.																												
7 a.m.																												
8 a.m.																												
9 a.m.																												
10 a.m.																												
11 a.m.																												
12 noon																												
1 p.m.																												
2 p.m.																												
3 p.m.																												
4 p.m.																												
5 p.m.																												
6 p.m.																												

How Well Do You Know Your Body?

Mom	**Partner**
When I am tense or under stress, I feel tension in my	When I am tense or under stress, I feel tension in my

Mom

When I am tense or under stress, I feel tension in my
- _____ head
- _____ jaws
- _____ neck
- _____ shoulders
- _____ chest
- _____ stomach
- _____ back
- _____ other _____

My body reacts to tension by
- _____ sweating
- _____ heart rate increasing
- _____ heart pounding
- _____ difficulty catching breath
- _____ clammy skin
- _____ trembling hands or legs
- _____ "butterflies" in stomach
- _____ nausea
- _____ gripping fists
- _____ itching/scratching
- _____ pumping top leg when legs crossed
- _____ biting nails
- _____ grinding teeth
- _____ speech difficulties
- _____ other _____

I can recognize signs of tension in my body by
_____
_____

I can prevent tension from overwhelming me by
_____
_____

I use the following calming techniques when needed
- _____ paced breathing
- _____ consciously relaxing all muscle groups
- _____ imagery
- _____ other _____

To cope with pain, I
- _____ need quiet to tune into myself
- _____ need to think about something else
- _____ need someone to be with me
- _____ need to talk with someone
- _____ need to be doing something
- _____ want help from a medical person
- _____ want to be alone
- _____ other _____

Partner

When I am tense or under stress, I feel tension in my
- _____ head
- _____ jaws
- _____ neck
- _____ shoulders
- _____ chest
- _____ stomach
- _____ back
- _____ other _____

My body reacts to tension by
- _____ sweating
- _____ heart rate increasing
- _____ heart pounding
- _____ difficulty catching breath
- _____ clammy skin
- _____ trembling hands or legs
- _____ "butterflies" in stomach
- _____ nausea
- _____ gripping fists
- _____ itching/scratching
- _____ pumping top leg when legs crossed
- _____ biting nails
- _____ grinding teeth
- _____ speech difficulties
- _____ other _____

I can recognize signs of tension in my body by
_____
_____

I can prevent tension from overwhelming me by
_____
_____

I use the following calming techniques when needed
- _____ paced breathing
- _____ consciously relaxing all muscle groups
- _____ imagery
- _____ other _____

To cope with pain, I
- _____ need quiet to tune into myself
- _____ need to think about something else
- _____ need someone to be with me
- _____ need to talk with someone
- _____ need to be doing something
- _____ want help from a medical person
- _____ want to be alone
- _____ other _____

Fun and Fast Format for Feeling Fit and Flexible

Head to toe in 5 minutes or more.

This standing sequence may be done all at one time, or the various exercises may be spaced out through a day as you feel the need to stretch or unwind. Other stretches can be done sitting at a desk, riding in a car or plane, or even lying or sitting in bed. Add a walk around the block, a bike ride, swim, or other aerobic exercise to your daily routine.

You will feel better when you feel fit and flexible!

Remember to:

- Use slow, controlled movements when stretching; never bounce or jerk.
- Work to feel stretch, not pain.
- Hold a stretch from 20 seconds to a minute or more to benefit from it.
- Exhale as you go into the stretch, then breathe normally.
- Actively feel the stretch in your muscles, not joints.
- Feel the release of tension as you let go.

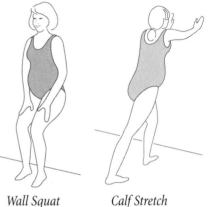

Wall Squat   *Calf Stretch*

Head and Neck

- Look far right; hold; center; far left; hold; center; repeat.
- Drop right ear to right shoulder; hold; drop left ear to left shoulder; hold; drop chin to chest; hold; repeat.

Shoulders, Arms, Hands

- Holding arms out shoulder level make small, then large circles in a spiral. Circle forward, then reverse.
- Lift elbows up to shoulder level with fingers and forearms pointing down; bending elbows, bring tightened fists in towards face; then straighten elbows, stretching arms and fingers out shoulder level. Repeat in and out picturing your arms as windshield wipers.

Abdominals, Back, Pelvic Floor

- Wall Stretch – step back against wall for wall stretch (page 17). "Hands up" position.
- Standing Pelvic Tilt – Tilt pelvis as you tighten abdominals (page 16).
- Add Kegel during tilt (page 18).

Legs

- Wall Squat – squat down; hold to feel tension in thighs; breathe through "pain" (page 17).
- Calf Stretch – turn to face wall; stretch (page 17)

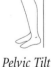

Wall Stretch   *Pelvic Tilt*

Feet

- Ankle Rotation – Hold on to wall or partner if needed for support and lift foot for ankle rotation.
- Standing foot stretch (do not curl toes). Pull ball of foot toward heel, raising arch. Release, repeat.

Body Stretch with Posture Check

- Stand tall dropping shoulders with arms at your side, then raise both arms straight overhead and stretch; lower arms to shoulder level, palms facing up; then, press arms back 5 times, pinching shoulder blades together with each press. Replace arms to your sides.
- Rub hands together to warm; place hands over eyes; rock gently forward and back on your feet until you "settle." Remove hands from eyes; drop shoulders, hands at side. Feel your body's posture. Relax head, eyes, jaws, shoulders, chest (big relaxing breath), release abdominal muscles, hips; feel tension flow all the way out your toes.
- Open eyes; feel refreshed, flexible, and "in line."

Nutrition Crossword Puzzle

ACROSS

1. You can easily combine grains and vegetables into a hearty _____.
3. Because vitamins B and C are not stored by the body, how often do you need to consume them?
5. Especially in pregnancy, it is dangerous to eat meat that is too _____.
6. A tropical orange fruit high in vitamins A and D, folate, and potassium
7. The "almost perfect" food that supplies protein, calcium, phosphorus, and vitamin D.
8. In addition to water, a recommended beverage.
9. A high-protein fish considered very safe for pregnant women.
10. Vitamin D supplements are recommended, especially for those who are rarely out in the _____.
11. Nutrition for the pregnant woman is especially important in the last three months of pregnancy because critical development is taking place in the baby's _____.
12. A handful of _____ is a healthy snack high in protein, fiber, and many minerals.
14. The factor which many believe may contribute MOST to the development of a healthy baby.
16. For heart-healthy eating, choose this kind of milk.
17. For safe eating, ____ fresh fruits and vegetables thoroughly before eating.
21. A seasoning many *wrongly* believe should be restricted during pregnancy.
22. For heart-healthy eating, choose this kind of meat, poultry, or fish.
23. Adding nuts, raisins, and whole grains to _____ dough can make these a healthier snack.
25. Amount of yogurt that counts as one cup in the Milk Group is _____ ounces.
28. Beans, nuts, whole grains and dairy products can be combined to provide protein sources which could substitute for _____.
29. Weight gain of approximately _____ pound(s) per week during the last three months of pregnancy is(are) recommended.
30. When eating "fast-foods," include a _____ with your meal to add valuable nutrients.

DOWN

2. A pregnant woman needs 60 grams of _____ each day.
3. Thiamin, a B vitamin, is called the "morale vitamin" because a deficiency may cause _____.
4. Liver; dairy products; dark-green, orange and deep _____ vegetables are excellent sources of vitamin A.
13. A nursing mother is encouraged to drink water and other liquids to _____.
15. Fruits and vegetables provide the most nutrients when eaten _____ or steamed.
18. A meal with broccoli, cheese sauce, canned salmon, and milk is very high in this mineral.
19. Green leafy vegetables and dry beans are the best sources of this important B vitamin, an essential component of blood cells.
20. This nutrient can be added to foods or eaten alone to add fiber to your diet.
21. Babies who are exposed to _____ in the womb are more likely to be born prematurely.
23. Green peppers, tomatoes, broccoli, strawberries, and _____ fruits are good sources of vitamin C.
24. The type of feeding recommended by the American Academy of Pediatrics for babies for the first year of life.
26. The body's demand for this mineral during pregnancy is so high that it is difficult to meet the daily requirement by diet alone.
27. Drinking _____ inhibits the absorption of iron from food eaten at the same meal.

Protein and Calorie Counter

Dairy Products:	Protein(g)	Calories
Butter, 1 tbsp.	Trace	102
Margarine, 1 tbsp.	Trace	101
†Milk:		
Whole, 1 cup	8	150
Skim, 1 cup	8	86
†Cheese:		
Cheddar, 1 oz.	7	114
American, 1 oz.	6	105
Cottage, creamed, ½ cup	13	108
Cream, 1 oz.	2	98
Swiss, 1 oz.	8	105
†Yogurt, fruit, lowfat, 1 cup	9	240
Vanilla Ice Cream, ½ cup	2	140
Vanilla Shake (Burger King)	9	321

Meat, Poultry, Fish, Eggs:	Protein(g)	Calories
Beef:		
Chuck, pot roast, 3 oz.	22	278
Hamburger, 75% lean, 3 oz.	21	235
Hamburger, 90% lean, 3 oz.	21	173
Roast, lean, 3 oz.	23	209
Steak, sirloin, lean, 3 oz.	26	180
Steak, round, lean, 3 oz.	24	165
Corned, 3 oz.	15	213
Stew, with vegetables, 1 cup	16	218
Chicken:		
Breast, roasted, 3½ oz.	29	193
Breast, fried, 3½ oz.	31	218
Thigh, skinless, roasted, 3 oz.	21	177
Duck, 3 oz.	16	286
Eggs, one	6	79
Fish:		
Haddock, fried, 3 oz.	16	194
Cod, poached	28	95
Shrimp, broiled, 3 oz.	18	84
Tuna, packed in water, 3 oz.	23	110
California roll	9	255
Lamb:		
Chop, broiled, 3 oz.	24	159
✓ Liver:		
Beef, 3 oz.	21	137
Chicken, 3 oz.	21	133
Pork:		
Bacon, crisp, 2 slices	4	72
Chop, 3 oz.	25	301
Ham steak, lean, 3 oz.	17	105
Ham, luncheon meat, 1 slice	5	52
Hot dog, one	5	144
Sausage, 1 piece	12	200
Turkey, light, 3 oz.	24	167
Turkey, hotdog	6	102
Veal:		
Cutlet, broiled, 3 oz.	23	185

Nuts and Seeds:	Protein(g)	Calories
†Almonds, 1 oz.	4	165
✓ Peanuts, 1 oz.	8	162
Peanut butter, 2 tbsp.	9	190
Pecans, 1 oz.	2	185
✓ Sunflower seeds, 1 oz.	5	163

✓ Dried Beans:	Protein(g)	Calories
Lima, cooked, ½ cup	7	108
Navy, cooked, ½ cup	8	112
Kidney, canned, ½ cup	7	102

Grains (✓Whole & fortified grains are high in folic acid.)	Protein(g)	Calories
Biscuits, one	2	103
Bread: white or wholewheat, 1 slice	2	65
Cereal, oatmeal, 1 oz.	5	110
Cereal, Rice Krispies, 1 oz.	2	110
Pasta (rotini), 2 oz.	7	210
Rice, brown, ½ cup	2½	108
Rice, white, ½ cup	2	85
Rolls, dinner, one	2	85
Cornbread, one	4	198
Saltines, five	1	52

Vegetables:	Protein(g)	Calories
✓ Asparagus, cooked, ½ cup	2	22
✓†Broccoli*, cooked, ½ cup	2	23
✓ Brussels sprouts*, cooked, ½ cup	2	30
†Cabbage*:		
Coleslaw, 1 serving	2	119
Cooked, ½ cup	1	16
Carrots, raw, ½ cup	1	31
Corn, cooked, ½ cup	3	89
✓ Edamame, ½ cup	11	125
✓ Green beans, cooked, ½ cup	1	22
Lettuce, leaf, ½ cup	1	5
✓ Lima beans, cooked, ½ cup	7	94
✓ Peas, cooked, ½ cup	3	67
Pepper, bell*, chopped, ½ cup	Trace	19
✓ Potatoes*:		
Baked (with skin on*) 1 medium	5	218
French fries, 10	2	158
Mashed, ½ cup	2	111
Chips, 1 oz.	2	150
✓†Spinach*, cooked, ½ cup	3	21
Tomato*, raw, 1 medium	1	24

Fruits:	Protein(g)	Calories
Apple, 1 medium	Trace	81
✓ Avocado, ½ large	2	153
Banana, 1 medium	1	109
✓ Cantaloupe*, ½ medium	2	90
Grapefruit*, ½	1	38
Grapes, Concord ½ cup	Trace	29
✓Orange*, 1 medium	1	62
✓†Orange juice*, 1 cup (calcium fortified)	2	112
Peach, fresh, 1 medium	1	37
Pear, fresh, 1 medium	1	97
Pineapple, fresh, ½ cup	Trace	38
Plum, 1 medium	1	36
Prune juice, 1 cup	2	182
Raisins, ½ cup	0	217
✓Strawberries*, raw, 1 cup	1	45
Watermelon, diced, ½ cup	1	26

Beverages (other):	Protein(g)	Calories
Coffee, black, 6 oz.	0	11
Beer, 12 oz.	1	146
Wine, red, 3½ oz.	Trace	74
Whiskey, gin, rum, vodka, 1 oz.	0	105

Desserts and Sweets:	Protein(g)	Calories
Cake:		
Chocolate with icing, 1 slice	2	169
Angel food, 1 slice	4	143
Doughnut, plain, one	3	210
Pie:		
Apple, 1 slice	3	302
Custard, 1 slice	6	207

Fast Foods:	Protein(g)	Calories
Subway 6-inch Turkey Sandwich	18	280
McDonald's Quarter Pounder	24	410
McDonald's Filet-O-Fish	15	380
Long John Silver's fish, 1 piece	12	260
KFC, grilled chicken breast	35	180
Pizza Hut cheese pizza –		
½ of 10" pie (thin crust)	25	450
Taco Bell taco, crunchy	7	150
Burger King french fries, medium	5	480
McDonald's Egg McMuffin	18	300

Vegetarian Choices:	Protein(g)	Calories
✓ Tofu (firm), 4 oz.	9	79
Tempeh, 4 oz.	21	223
Soy Milk, 8 oz.	10	140
Hummus, 2 tbsp.	2	50
Soup:		
✓ Split pea, 1 cup	9	164
Cream of broccoli, 1 cup	7	140
Vegetable, 1 cup	4	122

*Good sources of vitamin C   †Foods high in calcium   ✓Foods high in folic acid

Diet Evaluation

Become aware of your eating habits now, as the two of you will be setting the eating patterns in your home for years to come. Use this form to check your diet for any 24-hour period to be sure you are getting the recommended amount from each of the food groups. List all foods, including snacks. The amount of food needed will vary depending on your ages and activity levels, and the trimester of pregnancy for mom. See <www.choosemyplate.gov>. Moms click on "pregnancy and breastfeeding" and partners click on "general population." This online tool gives you information on your diet and links to nutrient information. You can receive an overall diet evaluation and may track what you eat up to a year. The servings listed below are for a 25 year-old pregnant woman who exercises 30 to 60 minutes a day. Her calorie needs vary from 2200 calories in the first trimester to 2600 in the third trimester.

Mother-To-Be/Nursing Mother	Breakfast	Lunch	Dinner	Snacks	Totals
					Basic food group servings:
					Grains (7 to 9 oz.) ____
					Vegetables (3 to 3 ½) ____
					Fruits (2 cups) ____
					Dairy (3 cups) ____
					Protein (6 to 6 ½ oz.) ____
					Oils (6 to 8 tsp.) ____
					Water (To thirst) ____
					Grams of protein:
					Calories:

Partner	Breakfast	Lunch	Dinner	Snacks	Totals
					Basic food group servings:
					Grains (6 to 8 oz.) ____
					Vegetables (2 ½ to 3 cups) ____
					Fruits (2 cups) ____
					Dairy (3 cups) ____
					Protein (5 ½ to 6 ½ oz.) ____
					Oils (6 to 8 tsp.) ____
					Water (To thirst) ____
					Grams of protein:
					Calories:

General Guidelines – Sixty grams of protein each day are recommended for pregnant women. Determine your own calorie needs and serving sizes at <choosemyplate.gov>. Two hundred extra calories are needed for breastfeeding mothers. The recommended number of calories for men ages 19 to 60 varies from 2200 to 3000 depending on age and physical activity.

Progressive Tense/Release Practice

By practicing the following tension-awareness exercise, you will learn to recognize tension as it builds in your body throughout the day. By listening to your body you may be able to release that tension before it turns to pain.

For each part of your body:

- First, think about how the muscle group feels now.
- Then, tighten – contract or stretch the muscle group; and
- Hold to a count of 5 as you concentrate on what you feel; study the sensation when the muscle is tight.
- Finally, release the tension to a count of 10, let go; compare the difference between feelings of tension and release.

Muscle	Tighten or Stretch	Hold & Concentrate	Release/Relax
Forehead	Raise eyebrows	Hold to a count of 5 & concentrate	Let go, release
	Frown	Hold to a count of 5 & concentrate	Smooth the forehead
Eyes	Look up, down, right, left	Hold to a count of 5 & concentrate	Close eyes softly
Mouth	Press lips together	Hold to a count of 5 & concentrate	Part lips slightly
	Smile (exaggerate)	Hold to a count of 5 & concentrate	Soften smile
	Press tongue against teeth	Hold to a count of 5 & concentrate	Let tongue feel thick
Jaws	Bite teeth together gently	Hold to a count of 5 & concentrate	Let jaw fall open slightly
	Drag jaw down, wide open	Hold to a count of 5 & concentrate	Close jaw softly
Neck	Pull head into shoulders like a turtle	Hold to a count of 5 & concentrate	Rotate head on neck
Shoulders	Round shoulders forward	Hold to a count of 5 & concentrate	Release to neutral
	Pull shoulders back	Hold to a count of 5 & concentrate	Release to neutral
	Pull shoulders down toward feet	Hold to a count of 5 & concentrate	Release to neutral
Arms	Pull tight against body	Hold to a count of 5 & concentrate	Allow to dangle
Hands	Clench fists	Hold to a count of 5 & concentrate	Allow fingers to curl gently
	Stretch fingers long	Hold to a count of 5 & concentrate	Release the stretch
Chest	Fill lungs with air	Hold to a count of 5 & concentrate	Let the air out
Abdomen	Pull belly in to hug baby	Hold to a count of 5 & concentrate	Let go of hug
Hips	Pinch buttocks together	Hold to a count of 5 & concentrate	Let muscles spread
Thighs	Push feet and legs together	Hold to a count of 5 & concentrate	Let them flop open
	Press hips and knees outward	Hold to a count of 5 & concentrate	Let them go loose
Legs	Flex foot and stretch leg	Hold to a count of 5 & concentrate	Drop foot and leg
Feet	Curl toes gently (do not point)	Hold to a count of 5 & concentrate	Release the curl

Sequence for Learning Progressive Relaxation

1. Progressive tense/release as outlined above.
2. Just think of each muscle listed above, then release that muscle without first tightening or stretching.
3. Think and release in larger groups all at one time:

    head, neck, shoulders, arms…release

    chest, abdomen, back…release

    hips, legs, feet…release

4. Final mastery is when you simply say to yourself, "let go" or "release" and your entire body relaxes!

Relaxing Words

Phrases to Relax With

This is a modified autogenic exercise

I feel very calm and quiet. I close my eyes and focus my awareness inside myself. I deepen my breathing and quiet my thoughts. I let my body be still and my muscles release.

My scalp is loose and relaxed. My head feels comfortable and quiet. My eyes feel heavy. My mouth smiles gently as my lips release. My tongue feels thick and moist. My cheeks are loose and my jaw droops. My face and my forehead are smooth, quiet, comfortable, and very relaxed. My neck is comfortable and still. My shoulders hang loose. My arms are floating and tingling. My fingers are curled and warm. My lungs breathe deeply, slowly, as my chest rises and falls with no effort, no thinking. My body just breathes for me; my heartbeat is strong and regular. My belly is soft, round, and filled with quiet energy. My baby inside is floating and peaceful, strong and healthy, warm, safe, and secure. My hips are loose. My legs are loose, motionless. I feel warmth flowing down into my feet. My legs, knees, and ankles are heavy and loose. Within the center of myself I feel quiet, calm, and peaceful. My baby feels my calmness and shares it.

Positive Affirmations

Every day my baby grows stronger and stronger.

I feel calm and at peace with the world.

I breathe energy into my baby.

My baby gives me strength to labor.

My world is safe and secure.

My body is made to give birth.

I am strong and able to birth my baby.

_____

_____

_____

_____

_____

_____

Words That Are Relaxing to Me

Circle the words you like

loose	free
limp	drained
warm	weak
cool	lax
heavy	rested
light	flabby
floating	slack
tingling	comfy
sagging	cozy
thick	secure
curled	snug
soft	mellow
whole	droopy
peaceful	quiet
calm	flexible
flaccid	_____
relaxed	_____
released	_____

Fill in Relaxing Words You Like to Describe

head _____

eyes _____

tongue _____

mouth _____

jaw _____

shoulders _____

arms _____

hands _____

fingers _____

chest _____

belly _____

baby _____

hips _____

legs _____

feet _____

Relaxing Images

Choose Your Own Journey

When you choose your own journey you are totally in control of your images and thoughts. Fill in the following blanks to record scenes, sensations, and suggestions that are pleasant and relaxing for you. Your journey may be to any real or imaginary place. Pretend that you take with you a magic bag that holds anything you need for your comfort.

Where will you go on this journey? _____ When you arrive what do you see? _____ The air around you feels _____ You are dressed very comfortably in _____ Notice the colors around you. What colors do you see? _____ Breathe in deeply and smell the fragrance of _____ in the air around you. Enjoy that scent that calms you and makes you feel safe, comfortable. As you walk around, what do you feel beneath your feet? _____ Is it soft, hard, crunchy, warm, cool? _____ What do you see in the distance? _____ What do you see nearby? _____ Is there something near you that you would like to touch, to feel, to experience? What is it like? _____ If you would like, you may touch it. Feel the texture, _____ the temperature, _____ the size, _____ and shape _____. What is the color? _____ Is there any water in your image? If so, use it to help you relax as you see fit. Is it just peaceful to look at or listen to, or do you wish to be in it, or touch it, or to drink from it? _____ Water cools and refreshes. Enjoy water by taste or by sight if it fits into your image. Food and drink are comforting. If you feel like it, you can reach into your magic bag and bring out whatever you would like to eat or drink. You may set a feast in your image or simply sip or snack. What would you have? _____ _____ If you choose to eat or drink, what will it be? _____ Focus on the taste: sweet or savory, _____ the texture: juicy or crisp, _____ the temperature: hot or cold _____. Enjoy!

Now find a special place in your image to lie down. Any props you may need are in your magic bag. Snuggle down, curl up, or stretch out to relax. Feel the sensation of total peace come over your entire body. Listen to the sounds around you. Look at the peaceful scene. Enjoy the colors, the textures you see and touch. Breathe in the calm, refreshing air. Tune in to this feeling. Remember it. You can come back to it at any time.

My Journey – *use the preceding suggestions to help you write your own very special and quieting journey.*

_____

_____

_____

_____

_____

_____

_____

_____

After you describe your journey, find a comfortable place to replay it in your mind. Allow the tension to leave your body as your breathing becomes slow and rhythmical and you transport yourself to your special place. The images you have designed will come alive in your mind and your body will relax. As you conclude your image, begin to move your relaxed body slowly. Take your time returning to full activity. When you do, you will have renewed energy, and a sense of well being.

The more you work with your journey, the faster you can achieve your relaxed state even in distracting and less than comfortable situations. Share your images with your partner so he or she can give you these comforting suggestions during your labor.

Practice Rhythmic Breathing

When either a true contraction or a practice contraction begins,

- take a cleansing breath,
- establish a focal point, and
- begin rhythmic breathing.

Breathe in one or more of the following ways through the contraction:

- inhale through nose…exhale out through mouth
- in through nose…out through nose
- in through mouth…out through mouth

Slow Breathing

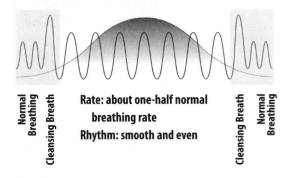

Rate: about one-half normal breathing rate
Rhythm: smooth and even

During a contraction:

- the scene or color I like to visualize is _____
- the phrase I like to say to myself is _____
- the most comfortable number to count to is _____

Breathing Patterns

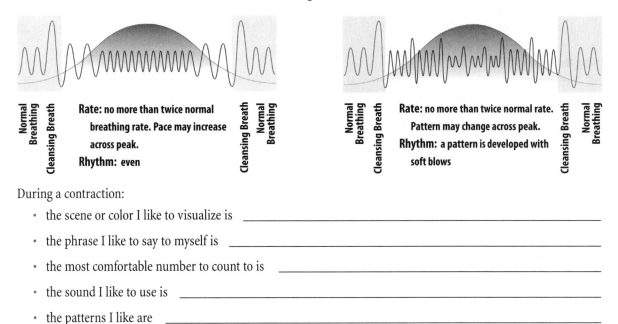

Rate: no more than twice normal breathing rate. Pace may increase across peak.
Rhythm: even

Rate: no more than twice normal rate. Pattern may change across peak.
Rhythm: a pattern is developed with soft blows

During a contraction:

- the scene or color I like to visualize is _____
- the phrase I like to say to myself is _____
- the most comfortable number to count to is _____
- the sound I like to use is _____
- the patterns I like are _____

With This Birth, I Plan to Try

Distractions

_____ Sleep and/or rest
_____ Take a walk
_____ Talk with family and friends
_____ Read
_____ Play a game
_____ Eat a light meal
_____ Breathe in patterns

Relaxation techniques

_____ Use slow breathing
_____ Consciously release each muscle group
_____ Release to partner's touch and/or massage
_____ Use visual imagery

Using the sense of vision

_____ External focal point
_____ Internal focal point

Using the sense of hearing

_____ Play music
_____ Talk
_____ Sing
_____ Read aloud
_____ Moan
_____ Pray
_____ Chant

Using the sense of smell

_____ Pillowcase from home
_____ Washcloth from home
_____ Favorite lotion or fragrance
_____ Aromatherapy

Using the sense of taste

_____ Popsicles
_____ Clear liquids such as juice, broth, tea, sports drinks
_____ Sour sucker
_____ Toothpaste and/or mouthwash

Using the sense of touch through temperature

_____ Ice
_____ Heating pad
_____ Hot water bottle
_____ Alternating hot/cold packs
_____ Warmed blankets
_____ Socks
_____ Warm bath and/or shower

Using the sense of touch through movement

_____ Walk
_____ Change positions frequently
_____ Stand
_____ Rock
_____ Hug someone
_____ Slow dance
_____ Do pelvic rock/tilt in all positions
_____ Use patterned breathing
_____ Gently shake joints
_____ Use rhythmical movements
_____ Use the "birth ball" for positioning and movement

Using the sense of touch through steady pressure

_____ Apply lip balm
_____ Kiss
_____ Maintain pressure on upper lip with index finger
_____ Use palms to squeeze something
_____ Stand on something hard
_____ Have someone do acupressure
_____ Apply pressure to the external genitalia (sit on a birth ball

Using the sense of touch on the skin

_____ Lightly stroke sheets with fingertips
_____ Feel partner's face with fingertips
_____ Do firm stroking on your belly
_____ Have partner do firm stroking on your belly
_____ Partner do gentle touch relaxation

Using the sense of touch through deep pressure and vibration

_____ Sit in a hot tub
_____ Use a shower massage
_____ Use a hot tub foot massager
_____ Use vibrating pillows
_____ Use a vibrating massager
_____ Have someone do acupressure
_____ Partner to massage (heavy pressure)

Other

_____ Partner + additional support person(s)
_____ Doula (professional labor support person)

_____

_____

_____

_____

_____

_____

What Helps Me Relax Best

Mom

Partner

The Kind of Touch or Massage I Like

Mom

Partner

Breathing Strategies I Like

Mom

Partner

The Kind of Music I Like

Mom

Partner

Pain Medications Preference Scale

Both the pregnant woman and her labor partner should understand her wishes for pain control in labor. Each of you choose the number that best matches your feelings, then compare. If your numbers are not very close, talk about your reasons. The pregnant woman's preferences are more important, but it helps build teamwork if you understand each other's concerns. The right hand column describes what kind of help she needs from her support people.

What It Means	How The Partner, Doula, and Caregiver Help
+10 She wants to feel nothing; desires anesthesia before labor begins.	An impossible extreme. If she has no interest in helping herself in labor, she needs to know she will have pain, and needs reassurance. She should discuss her wishes with her caregiver.
+9 Fear of pain; lack of confidence that she will be able to cope; dependence on staff for pain relief.	Help her accept that she will have some pain. Suggest she discuss fears with caregiver or childbirth educator. She needs information and reassurance, without false expectations.
+7 Definite desire for anesthesia as soon in labor as the doctor will allow it, or before labor becomes painful.	Be sure the caregiver is aware of her desire for early anesthesia and that she knows the potential risks. Learn whether this is possible in your hospital. Inform staff when you arrive.
+5 Desire for epidural anesthesia in active labor (4-5 cm); willingness to cope until then, perhaps with narcotic medication.	Encourage her in breathing and relaxation. Know comfort measures. Suggest medications to her in labor as she approaches active labor.
+3 Desire to use some pain medication, but wants as little as possible; plans to use self-help comfort measures for part of labor.	Plan to help her keep medication use low. Use comfort measures. Help her get medications when she wants them. Suggest reduced doses of narcotics or a "light and late" epidural block.
0 No opinion or preference. This is a rare attitude among pregnant women; but not uncommon among partners or support people.	Become informed. Discuss medications. Help her decide her preferences. If she has no preference ahead of time, follow her wishes during labor.
-3 Prefers that pain medications be avoided, but wants medication as soon as she requests it in labor.	Do not suggest that she take pain medications. Emphasize coping techniques. Do not try to talk her out of pain medications.
-5 Strong preference to avoid pain medications, mainly for benefit to baby and labor progress. Will accept medications for difficult or long labor.	Prepare yourself for a very active role. A doula will be most helpful for both the woman and partner. Know how to help her relax and use the breathing strategies. Know the comfort measures. Do not suggest medications. If she asks, interpret it as a need for more help and try different comfort measures and more intense emotional support first. You should, however, have a prearranged plan (e.g., a "last resort" code word) for how she can let you know she really has had enough and wants medication.
-7 Very strong desire for natural childbirth, for sense of personal gratification as well as to benefit baby and labor progress. Will be disappointed if she uses medications.	Follow the recommendations for -5, but with even greater commitment. This means planning not to use pain medications, unless complications develop that require painful procedures, or she is unable to respond to intensive labor support techniques for several contractions in a row. If she asks for medication, plan to encourage alternative comfort measures.
-9 Wants medication to be denied by staff, even if she asks for it.	This is very difficult for you – to be responsible for her satisfaction. Promise to help all you can, but help her realize the final decision is not yours. It is hers.
-10 Wants no medication, even for cesarean delivery.	An impossible extreme. Encourage her to learn of complications that require painful interventions. Help her get a realistic understanding of risks and benefits of pain medications.

Adapted from: *The Birth Partner* by Penny Simkin. Harvard Common Press. Reprinted with permission of the author.

Birth Options

Options to discuss with my partner and health care provider:	My ideal labor and birth would include:	If my ideal is not possible, I would like to:	If I need to have a cesarean birth, I would like to:
• Labor support (partner, other family, friend, doula)			
• Spontaneous labor or elective induction			
• Food and fluids by mouth			
• IV or heparin lock			
• Intermittent or continuous monitoring of the fetal heart tones			
• Movement and position changes: walking, slow dancing, rocking chair, birth ball			
• Warm bath/shower during labor			
• Use of comfort techniques: touch and massage, warm and cold packs, aromatherapy			
• Use of analgesia/anesthesia for pain relief			
• Spontaneous or directed pushing, choice of position			
• Perineal massage; routine episiotomy			
• Use of forceps, suction device			
• No separation of mother and baby after birth, or length of time with baby immediately after birth			
• Initiation of breastfeeding			
• Family/sibling visits—rooming in			
• Circumcision; anesthesia for circumcision			

Time Sharing

Mom

This pie represents 24 hours of your day. Draw wedges in the pie to show the number of hours you currently spend in each of your daily activities: eating, cooking, sleeping, at work, grooming, home maintenance/chores, leisure time for self, leisure time for couple, etc.

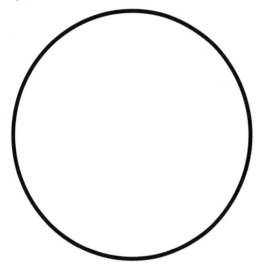

This pie represents 24 hours of your day after your baby arrives. Draw wedges in the pie to show the number of hours you think you will spend in each of your daily activities: eating, sleeping, cooking, at work, grooming, home maintenance/chores, leisure time for self, leisure time for couple, etc. *plus* time spent for baby feeding, diapering, laundry, consoling, etc.

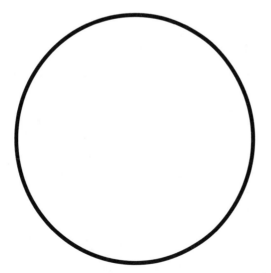

Dad

This pie represents 24 hours of your day. Draw wedges in the pie to show the number of hours you currently spend in each of your daily activities: eating, cooking, sleeping, at work, grooming, home maintenance/chores, leisure time for self, leisure time for couple, etc.

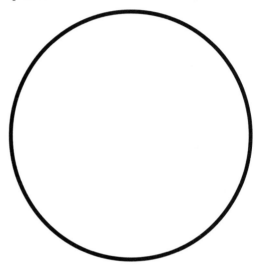

This pie represents 24 hours of your day after your baby arrives. Draw wedges in the pie to show the number of hours you think you will spend in each of your daily activities: eating, sleeping, cooking, at work, grooming, home maintenance/chores, leisure time for self, leisure time for couple, etc. *plus* time spent for baby feeding, diapering, laundry, consoling, etc.

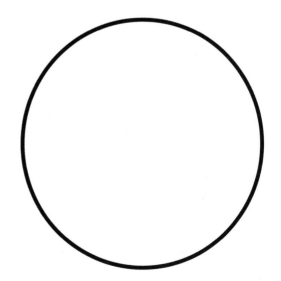

Puzzle Page

Match the following "problems of pregnancy" to the appropriate "comfort measures." Some may have more than one correct answer.

If you have:

1. leg cramps
2. back-ache
3. incontinence
4. swelling
5. heartburn
6. fatigue
7. constipation
8. hemorrhoids

Then you might try:

a. eat bran/drink water
b. rest/naps
c. calf stretches
d. Kegel exercise
e. sit, swim, or walk in water
f. small, frequent meals
g. posture and position
h. pelvic tilts

UNSCRAMBLE the following words for ideas of things to try in labor, then place the numbered letter in the appropriate boxes for more good advice!

SUMIC [_ _ _ _] (4)

HBAT [_ _ _ _] (16)

KLAW [_ _ _ _] (19)

DANTS [_ _ _ _ _] (15)

ROAASM [_ _ _ _ _ _] (10, 11)

TEHA [_ _ _ _] (9)

VLRFOSA [_ _ _ _ _ _ _] (1, 2)

SURREPSE [_ _ _ _ _ _ _ _] (18)

LARXE [_ _ _ _ _] (8)

HOSEWR [_ _ _ _ _ _] (21, 6)

CIE KACP [_ _ _   _ _ _ _] (3, 13)

GAMESI [_ _ _ _ _ _] (7)

KRCO [_ _ _ _] (17)

EECUNMNGORTAE [_ _ _ _ _ _ _ _ _ _ _ _ _] (22, 14, 20)

SAMGESA [_ _ _ _ _ _ _] (5, 12)

[_ _ _ _ _] , [_ _ _ _ _ _ _] , [_ _ _] [_ _ _ _ _ _ _]
1 2 3 4 5 , 6 7 8 9 10 11 12 , 13 14 15 16 17 18 19 20 21 22

Word Find:
Find and circle the ten words or phrases that may signal the onset of labor.

```
T O X V S C O N T R A C T I O N S H O
L B U Q R O A K L S N R W K L A E M T
J I K M U C U S P L U G D G Q U W R F
V O G U V F T L U X D M P O I S R L C
K C O H S W C R H V K Y E J O E N X R
N R U P T U R E O F M E M B R A N E S
D A J Z Q E V L F E Y B A C K A C H E
A M W F C K N P M S N E Q N V D O X R
G P A K D B D I A R R H E A Z W R K M
I S P S T O W Z N E S T I N G R I S W
P D U F N U M P I G T O J V D F H I L
```

Recommended Reading and Viewing for Pregnant Women and Their Families

Pregnancy

American College of Obstetricians and Gynecologists. 2005. *Your Pregnancy and Birth.*

Broder, Michael. 2004. *The Panic-Free Pregnancy.*

Kitzinger, Sheila. 2003. *The Complete Book of Pregnancy and Childbirth.*

National Geographic. 2006. *In the Womb* DVD.

Nilsson, Lennart. 2009. *A Child is Born.*

Simkin, Penny, April Bolding, Ann Keppler, Janelle Durham, & Janet Whalley. 2010. *Pregnancy, Childbirth and the Newborn.*

Childbirth

Davis, Elizabeth & Debra Pascali-Bonaro. 2010. *Orgasmic Birth: Your Guide To a Safe, Satisfying, and Pleasurable Birth Experience.*

Gaskin, Ina May. 2003. *Ina May's Guide to Childbirth.*

Harper, Barbara. 2005. *Gentle Birth Choices.*

Lake, Ricki & Abby Epstein. 2010. *Your Best Birth: Know All Your Options, Discover the Natural Choices, and Take Back the Birth Experience.*

Lamaze International. 2000. *Everyday Miracles (video clip).* View at no cost at <www.lamaze.org>. See "Additional Videos" on home page.

Lamaze International. 2009. *Lamaze Healthy Birth Practices: Healthy Birth Your Way* video clips and pamphlets. Available at no cost at <www.lamaze.org>.

Lothian, Judith & Charlotte DeVries. 2010. *The Official Lamaze Guide: Giving Birth with Confidence.* Visit the blog at <http://givingbirthwithconfidence.org/>.

Sundin, Juju & Sarah Murdoch. 2008. *JuJu Sundin's Birth Skills – Proven Pain Management Techniques for Your Labour and Birth.*

Doulas, Labor Support

Klaus, Marshall, Phyllis Klaus, & John Kennell. 2002. *The Doula Book.*

Simkin, Penny. 2008. *The Birth Partner.*

Stein, Elissa & Jon Lichtenstein. 2007. *Don't Just Stand There – How to Be Helpful, Clued-In, Supportive, Engaged, Meaningful, and Relevant in the Delivery Room.*

Nutrition

American Dietetic Association (ADA) & Elizabeth M. Ward. 2009. *Expect the Best: Your Guide to Healthy Eating Before, During, and After Pregnancy.*

Jones, Catherine & Rose Ann Hudson. 2009. *Eating for Pregnancy: The Essential Guide and Cookbook for Today's Mothers-to-be.*

Exercise

Butler, Joan Marie. 2006. *Fit & Pregnant.*

Clapp, James. 2002. *Exercising Through Your Pregnancy.*

Freedman, Francoise. 2004. *Yoga for Pregnancy, Birth, and Beyond.*

Noble, Elizabeth. 2003. *Essential Exercises for the Childbearing Year.*

Yoga Journal and Lamaze. 2004. *Yoga for Your Pregnancy* DVD. Order from <www.yogaforyourpregnancy.com>

Dads

Sears, Robert & James Sears. 2006. *Father's First Steps: 25 Things Every New Dad Should Know.*

Web It!

Multiples	Carter, Cindy, Jeanne Green, & Debby Amis. 2011. *Preparing for Multiples – The Family Way.*
	Gromada, Karen. 2007. *Mothering Multiples – Breastfeeding and Caring for Twins.*
	Leiter, Gila. 2000. *Everything You Need to Know to Have a Healthy Twin Pregnancy.*
	Noble, Elizabeth. 2003. *Having Twins.*
	Luke, Barbara & Tamara Eberlein. 2010. *When You're Expecting Twins, Triplets, or Quads.*
	Rudat, April. 2007. *Oh Yes You Can Breastfeed Twins…Plus More Tips for Simplifying Life with Twins.*
Breastfeeding	Behrmann, Barbara. 2005. *The Breastfeeding Café.*
	Colburn-Smith, Cate & Andrea Serrette. 2007. *The Milk Memos: How Real Moms Learned to Mix Business with Babies–and How You Can, Too.*
	Gaskin, Ina May. 2009. *Ina May's Guide to Breastfeeding.*
	The Healthy Children Project. 2011. *The Magical Hour – Holding Your Baby Skin to Skin in the First Hour After Birth* DVD. Order from <www.healthychildren.cc>.
	Huggins, Kathleen. 2010. *The Nursing Mother's Companion.*
	Mohrbacher, Nancy & Kathleen Kendall-Tacket. 2010. *Breastfeeding Made Simple.*
	Silverman, Andi. 2007. *Mama Knows Breast – A Beginner's Guide to Breastfeeding.*
	Wiessinger, Diane, Diana West, & Teresa Pitman. 2010. *The Womanly Art of Breastfeeding.*
Postpartum	Placksin, Sally. 2000. *Mothering the New Mother – Your Postpartum Resource Companion.*
Newborn Care	Caplan, Frank, ed. 1995. *The First Twelve Months of Life.*
	Jana, Laura A. & Jennifer Shu. 2010. *Heading Home With Your Newborn: From Birth to Reality.* (Published by the American Academy of Pediatrics.)
	Klaus, Marshall & Phyllis Klaus. 2000. *Your Amazing Newborn.*
	Leach, Penelope. 2010. *Your Baby and Child: From Birth to Age Five.*
	McKenna. James. 2007. *Sleeping with Your Baby – A Parent's Guide to Cosleeping.*
	Sears, William & Martha Sears. 2003. *The Baby Book: Everything You Need to Know About Your Baby from Birth to Age Two.*
	Teddler, Jan. 2009. *H.U.G.* DVD. Order from <www.hugyourbaby.com/order.html>.
Parenting	Clarke, Jean Illsley. 1998. *Growing Up Again.*
	Faber, Adele & Elaine Mazlish. 1999. *How to Talk So Kids Will Listen and Listen So Kids Will Talk.*
	Nugent, Kevin. 2011. *Your Baby is Speaking to You: A Visual Guide to the Amazing Behaviors of Your Newborn and Growing Baby.*
	Sears, William & Martha Sears. 2001. *The Attachment Parenting Book.*
	Siegel, Daniel & Mary Hartzell. 2004. *Parenting from the Inside Out.*
Evidence-Based Information on Cesarean Birth	Childbirth Connection. 2006. *What Every Pregnant Woman Needs to Know about Cesarean Birth.* Available for no cost at <www.childbirthconnection.org>.
Controversies in Maternity Care	Block, Jennifer. 2008. *Pushed: The Painful Truth About Childbirth and Modern Maternity Care.*
	Gaskin, Ina May. 2011. *Birth Matters.*

Childbirth Organizations and Resources

Lamaze International
Weekly pregnancy e-newsletter, safe and healthy birth videos and information, childbirth educator referrals and training

<www.lamaze.org>
Click on "New and Expectant Parents"
(800) 368-4404 or (202) 367-1128

International Childbirth Education Association (ICEA)
Childbirth educator referrals and training, bookstore

<www.icea.org>
(612) 854-8660
ICEA Bookstore (800) 624-4934

Childbirth and Postpartum Professional Organization (CAPPA)
Childbirth educator referrals and training

<www.cappa.net>
(888) MY-CAPPA

Childbirth Connection
Evidence-based information on pregnancy and birth

<www.childbirthconnection.org>
(212) 777-5000

Coalition for Improving Maternity Care Services (CIMS)
Information about mother-friendly childbirth

<www.motherfriendly.com>
(888) 282-CIMS or (904) 285-1613

The National Women's Health Information Center
General health information including pregnancy and birth

<www.4woman.gov>
(800) 994-9662

DONA International
Doula referrals and training information, books, massagers, comfort items for labor

<www.dona.org>
(888) 788-DONA

International Lactation Consultant Association (ILCA)
Referrals to lactation consultants

<www.ilca.org>
(919) 861-5577

La Leche League
Referrals to breastfeeding support groups, books, and other resources

<www.lalecheleague.org>
(708) 519-7730

Labor and Birth Questionnaire

Mail this questionnaire to your childbirth educator as soon as possible after birth

Your name _____

Partner's name _____

Baby's birthdate _____

Baby's name _____

Weight _____ Length _____ Sex _____

Number of children prior to this birth _____

Doctor/midwife present at the birth _____

Hospital/Birth Center _____

Dates of classes attended _____

Childbirth educator _____

Number of classes mother attended _____

Number of classes partner attended _____

How much time did you practice each week? _____

Picture of new baby or new family

Labor and Birth Experience

Type of birth: Vaginal _____   Cesarean birth _____

Was this a normal, full-term, uncomplicated pregnancy? Yes _____ No _____ If not, please explain _____

_____

Was labor induced? No _____ Yes _____   If yes, how? Medication to soften /ripen cervix _____; Pitocin _____;

By health care provider rupturing membranes_____

If labor was induced, what was the reason given for the induction? _____

How did you know that labor had begun? _____

If the birth was by cesarean, when were you told that a cesarean would have to be done? _____

What was the reason given for the cesarean? _____

_____

During labor, did the doctor rupture your membranes?   No _____ Yes _____

If yes, at approximately how many centimeters dilation? _____

Prior to birth, what was your rating on the "Pain Medications Preference Scale" (page 110)?_____

(continued on back)

How long did you labor at home? _____

What was the approximate length of labor? _____ Time spent pushing? _____

How many hours were you in the hospital before birth? _____

What medications were given during labor? _____

What medications were given during pushing? _____

How did you feel about these medications? _____

_____

Location of birth: Birthing room _____   Delivery room _____

Describe how you pushed. _____

Did you have an episiotomy? _____   Any tears of perineum? _____

Were forceps or a vacuum extractor used? _____   If yes, what was the reason? _____

Who was with you during labor? _____

Who was with you during the birth? _____

Describe briefly the type of guidance and support that you received from:

     Doctor/Midwife _____

     _____

     Nursing staff _____

     _____

     Labor partner _____

What were the positive parts of your birth experience? _____

_____

What were the negative parts of your birth experience? _____

_____

Were you able to keep your baby with you immediately after birth? _____   If yes, for how long? _____

Describe your feelings at that time. _____

Did you have rooming-in? _____

If rooming-in was not available, were you able to get your baby for frequent feedings? _____

How are you feeding your baby?   Breast _____   Formula _____

If the baby is a boy, did you have him circumcised?   No _____   Yes _____

Now that you have had a chance to use your knowledge, do you think any areas should have been stressed in greater detail? Include comments on class, class content, and/or instructor. _____

_____

If you could change any aspect of your birth experience, what would it be? _____

_____

What advice or recommendations do you have for couples having their babies at this hospital/birth center? _____

_____

Mother's Labor and Birth Summary

	What were you feeling? (physically and emotionally)	What helped you the most to cope?	What did your partner do that was helpful?	Comments or suggestions
Early Labor				
Active Labor				
Transition				
Pushing				
Postpartum				

May I share this questionnaire with future classes?   Yes _____   No _____

Labor Partner's Birth Report

Initially, how did you feel about taking the classes with your partner? _____
_____
_____
_____

Did your concerns about childbirth change as a result of the classes? _____
_____
_____
_____

As a labor partner, were you adequately prepared for this birth? _____
_____
_____
_____

What should have been covered more thoroughly in class? _____
_____
_____
_____

What specific problems did she have during labor, and what did you do to help? _____
_____
_____
_____

Was her labor what you expected? _____
_____
_____
_____

Were you with her during birth? _____ How did you feel? _____
_____
_____
_____

What suggestions would you give to other labor partners? _____
_____
_____
_____

Add any additional comments regarding course content, instructor, or hospital/birth center experience. _____
_____
_____
_____

Also Available from The Family Way

Preparing for Multiples – The Family Way

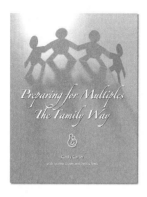

Designed especially for parents expecting twins, triplets, or more!

Prepárandose para la llegada de su bebé

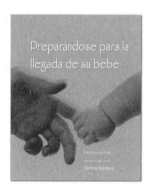

The Spanish adaptation of our handbook.

Especially for childbirth educators:
(Some posts and tweets may be of interest to expectant parents.)
Blog: www.thefamilyway.com
Twitter: http://twitter.com/thefamilyway

Contact us about bulk pricing for our handbook
and teaching resources for childbirth educators.

The Family Way Publications, Inc.

Phone:	(713) 528-0277
Fax:	(713) 583-6187
Website:	www.thefamilyway.com
E-mail:	info@thefamilyway.com